Pediatric CCRN Review Study Guide

By Stephanie Doig MS, BS, RN, CCRN

Pediatric CCRN Review Study Guide

by
Stephanie Doig MS, BS, RN, CCRN

Copyright © [2017] by [Stephanie Doig]
All rights reserved. No part of this book may be reproduced, scanned,
or distributed in any printed or electronic form without permission.
First Edition: [November 2017]
Printed in the United States of America

To my sweet, sweet husband Enrique and my dog Inti. Thank you for believing in me and supporting me during the time spent preparing this study guide.

Stephanie Doig

Table of Contents

Acknowledgement ix
Preface... xi
Chapter 1 Cardiovascular 1
Chapter 2 Pulmonary 9
Chapter 3 Endocrine/Hematology/Gastrointestinal/Renal/
Integumentary... 19
Chapter 4 Musculoskeletal/Neurology/Psychosocial 35
Chapter 5 Multisystem...49
Chapter 6 Professional Caring &Ethical Practice....................63
Chapter 7 Practice Question Answers................................69
References...85

Stephanie Doig

Acknowledgements

I gratefully acknowledge my fellow York College of Pennsylvania alumni Adam Poller for proposing this project and this study guide. Thank you for your guidance through the planning and development stages.

I would like to thank my PICU family at Inova Children's Hospital. I learned more than just how to be a great PICU nurse. The level of excellence expected daily is truly remarkable.

Thank you to Sara Knippen and Carol Rauen at American Association of Critical-Care Nurses (AACN) for providing guidance in the creation of test questions.

Stephanie Doig

Preface

This study guide is for use in conjunction with the Pediatric CCRN Review Course to assist nurses in obtaining pediatric CCRN certification. Obtaining pediatric CCRN certification seeks to promote improved outcomes in the care of critically ill children in pediatric intensive care units (PICUs).

Stephanie Doig

Chapter 1

I. Clinical Judgment:
A. Cardiovascular (15%) = 22.5 questions

1. ACUTE PULMONARY EDEMA

Acute pulmonary edema is defined as fluid in the air spaces of the lungs categorized into cardiac and non-cardiac causes. Cardiac causes include congestive heart failure (CHF), coronary artery disease, hypertension, heart valve disease, and reperfusion injury after cardiovascular surgery. Non-cardiac causes include near drowning, inhalation injury, and acute respiratory distress syndrome (ARDS). Pulmonary edema, pulmonary hemorrhage, overwhelming infection, aspiration pneumonitis, and pulmonary venous congestion manifest as perihilar opacities, radiopacity, and a generalized hazy appearance on chest x-ray.

Pulmonary edema in near-drowning patients is likely caused by acute myocardial depression secondary to increased left ventricular afterload, hypoxia, ARDS, interstitial fluid flux secondary to extreme negative pleural pressure generated by respiratory attempts with a closed glottis, and neurogenic causes. Neurogenic causes are unclear, but may be related to development of increased systemic and pulmonary artery pressure in response to intracranial hypertension.

Pulmonary edema may be seen 8-48 hours after an inhalation injury and is characterized by edema of the upper and lower airways, pulmonary interstitial edema, hypoxemia, and decreased lung compliance.

2. CARDIAC SURGERY (E.G., CONGENITAL DEFECTS)

Recovering a patient after cardiovascular surgery requires careful preparation to ensure emergency equipment is readily accessible and rapid assessment by the nurse of the child's baseline hemodynamic baseline. The nurse uses acute and frequent assessment techniques to rapidly obtain and note changes of status through physical exam, hemodynamic monitoring, and laboratory analysis.

Cardiac output is a product of heart rate and stroke volume. Stroke volume is affected by preload, afterload, and contractility. Preload is the pressure in the ventricle at end diastole. Afterload is resistance to ventricular ejection, which may result from increased pulmonary vascular resistance, systemic vascular resistance, or residual outflow tract obstruction.

1. An infant exhibits bradycardia after cardiac surgery. The nurse attributes which of the following as a cause?
a. Increased systemic vascular resistance
b. Decreased pulmonary vascular resistance
c. Increased contractility
d. Decreased ventricular compliance

(See Chapter 7 for answers)

3. CARDIAC/VASCULAR CATHETERIZATION

A. DIAGNOSTIC

B. INTERVENTIONAL

Cardiac catheterization interventions include device implantation (ASD/VSD occluders, PDA closure devices, coils, intravascular stents, and implantable valves), balloon dilation/valvuloplasty (performed for stenotic vessels and valves), radiofrequency ablation, and placement of surgical shunts to pulmonary arteries.

2. A baby who is recovering from a patent ductus arteriousus (PDA) closure develops shortness of breath and hematuria. The nurse anticipates
a. Return to the cath lab
b. Administration of platelets
c. A portable chest x-ray
d. Extracorporeal membrane oxygenation (ECMO)

4. CARDIOGENIC SHOCK

Cardiogenic shock is defined as impairment in cardiac function leading to failure in maintaining adequate tissue oxygenation. Compensatory mechanisms have deleterious effects. Compensatory mechanisms include the sympathetic nervous system, the renin-angiotensin-aldosterone system, nonosmotic release of arginine vasopressin, natriuretic hormone system, endothelial hormones, cytokines, ventricular dilation, ventricular hypertrophy, diastolic heart failure, and molecular basis for myocyte dysfunction.

5. CARDIOMYOPATHIES
A. DILATED
B. HYPERTROPHIC
C. IDIOPATHIC
D. RESTRICTIVE

Cardiomyopathy is defined as changes in the myocardium that produce ventricular dysfunction, decreased ventricular ejection fraction, increased myocardial mass, and myocyte degeneration. Cardiomyopathy may be dilated, hypertrophic, restrictive, or idiopathic in nature. Dilated cardiomyopathy accounts for at least half of cardiomyopathies.

3. End organ damage from dilated cardiomyopathy is caused by
a. Stiffness of the myocardium
b. Hypereosinophilic syndrome
c. Increased afterload and vasoconstriction
d. Increased release of intracellular calcium

5. DYSRHYTHMIAS

Dysrhythmias require the nurse to quickly assess the effect of the rhythm on the patient's hemodynamic status. Ninety percent of pediatric arrhythmias are supraventricular tachycardias. Other arrhythmias include bradyarrhythmias, rhythms originating in the sinus node, rhythms originating in the atria, rhythms originating in the AV junction, rhythms originating in the ventricles, and atrioventricular (AV) blocks.

4. Assessment findings of a patient's electrocardiogram (ECG) reveal a heart rate of 124 bpm with an inverted P-wave immediately

following each R-wave. The nurse anticipates which of the following?
a. Initiation of overdrive pacing
b. Synchronized cardioversion
c. Administration of potassium chloride
d. Administration of packed red blood cells

6. HEART FAILURE

Similar to cardiogenic shock, heart failure is an inability of the heart to meet the demands of the body. Heart failure is a spectrum, with no definitive point between severe congestive heart failure and shock. In children, congenital heart disease is the most common cause of heart failure. Signs and symptoms are categorized into an adrenergic response (tachycardia, tachypnea, cool skin, oliguria, and diaphoresis), systemic venous congestion (hepatomegaly, periorbital edema, ascites, and pulmonary effusion), pulmonary venous congestion (tachypnea, retractions, nasal flaring, and pulmonary edema), and nonspecific signs of cardiorespiratory distress (irritability, change in responsiveness, fatigue, poor feeding, and failure to thrive).

7. HYPERTENSIVE CRISIS

Hypertensive crisis is excessive blood pressure (BP) elevation that may lead to dysfunction of cerebral autoregulation, vasospasms, ischemia, increased capillary pressure and permeability, cerebral edema, and hemorrhage. It may be caused by renal parenchymal disease, neurologic dysfunction, pheochromocytoma, pituitary tumor, coarctation of the aorta, congenital adrenal hyperplasia, and Cushing syndrome.

8. MYOCARDIAL CONDUCTION SYSTEM DEFECTS

First-degree heart block is defined as prolonged conduction through the AV node producing a long PR interval. Second-degree heart block is an intermittent failure of conduction impulses from the atria to the ventricles. It is categorized into Mobitz type I and Mobitz type II. Third-degree heart block is a complete failure of atrial impulse conduction through the ventricles.

5. A child is noted to have a prolonged PR interval. The nurse suspects which of the following as the cause?
a. Systemic lupus erythmatosus
b. ASD closure
c. Hypermagnesemia
d. Hypoglycemia

9. STRUCTURAL HEART DEFECTS (ACQUIRED AND CONGENITAL, INCLUDING VALVULAR DISEASE)

Acyanotic defects result in systemic circulation shunting into pulmonary circulation. It is called a left to right shunt because blood on the left side of the heart (systemic) blood shunts to the right (pulmonary) side of the heart. These include patent ductus arteriosus (PDA), atrial septal defect (ASD), ventricular septal defect (VSD), atrioventricular septal defect (AVSD, aka AV Canal), and double outlet right ventricle (DORV).

Obstructive defects lead to obstruction of blood flow. Aortic stenosis, hypoplastic left heart syndrome (HLHS), coarctation of the aorta, mitral valve disease/mitral stenosis, congenital mitral insufficiency, and valvular pulmonary stenosis.

Cyanotic defects cause pulmonary blood shunting into systemic circulation, also known as a right to left shunt. These include Tetralogy of Fallot, transposition of the great arteries (TGA), tricuspid atresia (TAT), truncus arteriosus, total anomalous pulmonary venous return (TAPVR), and pulmonary atresia with intact ventricular septum (PA/IVS). Children with cyanotic defects should be permitted to have low sats because administering oxygen will not improve sats and may cause oxygen toxicity to the lungs.

6. The knee-to-chest position is appropriate treatment of cyanosis in which of the following patients?
a. Unrepaired congenital mitral stenosis
b. Unrepaired tetralogy of Fallot
c. Unrepaired AV canal
d. Unrepaired hypoplastic left heart syndrome

Stephanie Doig

Chapter 2

I. Clinical Judgment:
B. Pulmonary (16%) = 24 questions

1. ACUTE PULMONARY EMBOLUS

Acute pulmonary embolism (PE) is a major cause of death and complications after surgery. Presence of a central venous catheter also increases the risk of venous thromboembolism and possible PE. PE results in right ventricular failure. Right ventricular failure is the inability of the right ventricle to provide adequate blood flow through the pulmonary circulation at a normal central venous pressure. Obstructed flow through the pulmonary arteries leads to increased dead space (pulmonary vasculature that is oxygenated, but not perfused) which manifests as decreased end-tidal carbon dioxide (ETCO2).

2. ACUTE RESPIRATORY DISTRESS SYNDROME (ARDS), TO INCLUDE ACUTE LUNG INJURY (ALI) AND RESPIRATORY DISTRESS SYNDROME (RDS)

ARDS is respiratory failure due to diffuse alveolar-capillary membrane injury causing permeability or elevated protein pulmonary edema. Initial events leading up to lung injury include sepsis, pneumonia, and aspiration. Management may include high positive end expiratory pressure (PEEP) with low tidal volume, high frequency oscillation ventilation (HFOV), permissive hypercapnia, surfactant, prone positioning, and nitric oxide.

Respiratory acidosis occurs when CO2 levels rise high enough to lower the serum pH below 7.35. Increased CO2 can be the result of central nervous system depression, intrinsic airway disease, chest wall instability, a compromised diaphragm, compromised upper airway muscle function, or alveolar disease. Normal pH is 7.35-7.45 while normal pCO2 levels are 35-45 mmHg.

7. The function of surfactant is to
    a. Vasodilate the pulmonary vasculature
    b. Decrease pulmonary shunting
    c. Decrease viscosity of pulmonary secretions
    d. Prevent alveolar collapse at end expiration

(see Chapter 7 for answers)

3. ACUTE RESPIRATORY FAILURE

Respiratory failure is defined as exchange of oxygen and carbon dioxide (CO2) that is not sufficient to meet the demands of the body resulting in hypoxemia, hypercarbia (also known as hypercapnia), or both. Hypercarbia is PaCO2 > 50-75 mm Hg. Causes of respiratory failure include hypoventilation, ventilation of perfusion (V/Q) mismatch, diffusion abnormalities, and intrapulmonary shunting.

The oxyhemoglobin dissociation curve is a graph representing hemoglobin's affinity for oxygen. The partial pressure of oxygen is on the x-axis and oxygen saturation is on the y-axis. A shift to the right reflects hemoglobin with less affinity for oxygen while a shift to the left reflects hemoglobin reflects hemoglobin with more affinity for oxygen. Factors causing a shift to the right include acidosis, hypercapnia, and hyperthermia. Factors shifting the curve to the left include alkalosis, hypocapnia, and hypothermia.

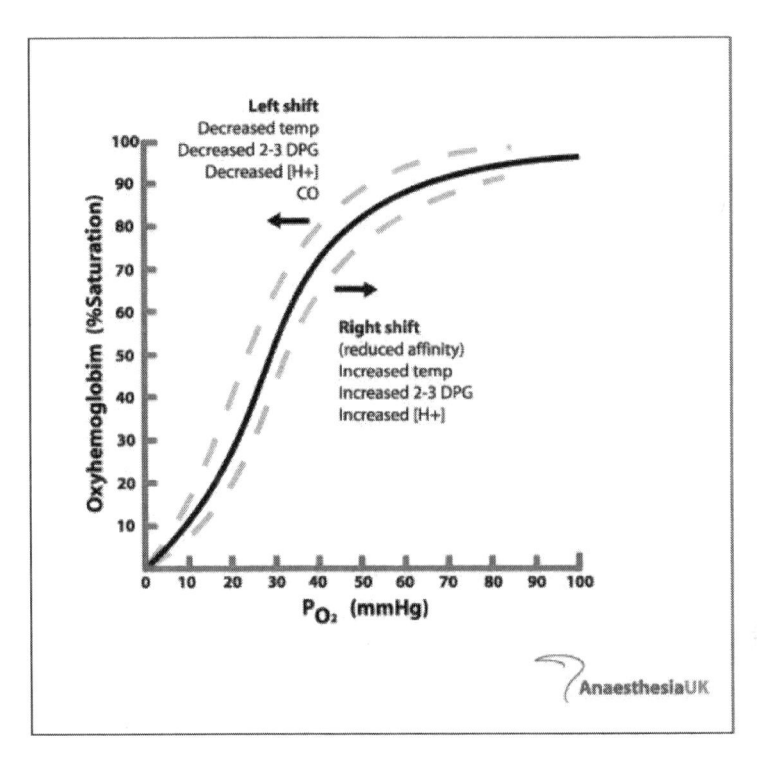

8. Interpret the following blood gas
   pH 7.50
   CO2 32 mmHg
   HCO3 31 mmol/L
   pO2 87
   a. Respiratory acidosis
   b. Respiratory alkalosis
   c. Metabolic acidosis
   d. Metabolic alkalosis

9. The nurse expects which of the following blood gas results in a child with a central nervous system disorder?

    a. Respiratory acidosis

    b. Respiratory alkalosis

    c. Metabolic acidosis

    d. Metabolic alkalosis

4. ACUTE RESPIRATORY INFECTION (E.G., PNEUMONIA)

Pneumonia is defined as inflammation of the lung parenchyma caused by infection (bacterial or viral), aspiration, chemical inhalation, or toxic agents. Bacterial pneumonia is characterized by high fever, sudden onset, cough, tachypnea, nasal flaring, cyanosis, crackles, change in behavior, anorexia, vomiting, diarrhea, and abdominal pain.

5. AIR-LEAK SYNDROMES

Air-leak syndromes include pneumothorax (air collection around the lung), pneumopericardium (air collection around the heart), and pneumomediastinum (air collection in the mediastinum). Mechanically ventilated patients receiving high tidal volumes and high pressures are at risk for air-leak syndromes because the elevated pressures push air out of the respiratory tract.

Chest tubes are used to evacuate air, fluid, chyle, or blood in air-leak syndromes. Vaseline dressings are not recommended for chest tubes while in place. Bubbling in the chamber may indicate a leak.

Chylothorax is the accumulation of lymph fluid in the chest as a result of injury to or obstruction of the thoracic duct or a large lymphatic vessel during cardiac surgery. Chylothorax is confirmed with presence of white or creamy lymphatic drainage in the chest tube. Treatment requires drainage of the lymph fluid by a chest tube or repeat thoracentesis. A medium-chain triglyceride diet may be recommended as well as the use of an octreotide infusion and surgical ligation of the thoracic duct.

6. ASPIRATION

Aspiration pneumonia is a group of disorders causing contamination of the lower airway with foreign material. Patients who aspirate may show no symptoms, mild symptoms, or the event may be acute and life threatening. Saliva, gastric contents, saline, water, barium, nasogastric feeds, and other contents may be aspirated. A life threatening aspiration event may produce direct injury to the mucosal surface of the respiratory tract, which can result in diffuse damage of the alveoli, hemorrhage, and necrotizing bronchiolitis.

7. BRONCHOPULMONARY DYSPLASIA

Bronchopulmonary dysplasia (BPD) is a chronic lung disease in premature infants leading to decreased lung compliance, increased airway resistance, severe expiratory flow limitations caused by airway edema, overinflation, and atelectasis.
Compliance is the relationship of volume and pressure within a closed space, such as the lung. It is determined by how elastic the lung is based on how much surfactant is present in the alveoli. Greater compliance (greater elasticity) will facilitate lower peak

inspiratory pressure (PIPs). Mean airway pressure is affected by multiple factors including tidal volume, PEEP, and PIP. PEEP may slightly impair carbon dioxide elimination because it slightly stents open the airway. CPAP provides positive airway pressure through both inspiration and expiration when the patient is breathing spontaneously. Patients with decreased lung compliance include patients with pneumonia, respiratory distress syndrome, fibrosis, and pulmonary edema.

8. CONGENITAL ANOMALIES (E.G., DIAPHRAGMATIC HERNIA, TRACHEOESOPHAGEAL FISTULA, CHOANAL ATRESIA, TRACHEOMALACIA, TRACHEAL STENOSIS)

Diaphragmatic hernia is a congenital defect or an acquired defect caused by trauma involving the diaphragm resulting in abdominal contents in the chest cavity.

Malacia comes from a Greek word meaning soft and is used to describe weakness or insufficiently rigid. Tracheomalacia results in collapsing of the part of the airway, resulting in stridor. Stridor is lessened when the patient is sleeping and breathing restfully.

Transesophageal fistula is an abnormal separation between the trachea and the esophagus. Fives types exist, depending on the location of the anomaly. Nursing management includes maintaining NPO status, managing IV hydration and fluid/electrolyte needs, maintaining the head of bed elevated, constant suctioning to keep the upper airway clear of secretions, preparation for surgical repair, and postoperative care. Complications include respiratory distress, aspiration, esophageal stricture, and anastomotic leak.

Choanal atresia is a rare congenital anomaly characterized by blocking of the nasopharynx. Signs and symptoms include intermittent cyanosis that resolves when the infant cries, unless the infant has learned to mouth breathe. Surgical intervention is necessary to correct the problem. Nursing intervention includes ensuring that the nasopharynx remains open. Inserting a nasogastric tube is the best way to ensure patency.

Tracheal stenosis is scarring and/or narrowing of the airway. Inflating the cuff with the minimal amount necessary to decrease irritation to the airway, monitoring endotracheal tube (ETT) cuff pressure every 8 hours, and suctioning above the cuff frequently can prevent tracheal stenosis. Treatment is aimed at keeping the airway from narrowing and may include surgical intervention and placement of a laryngeal stent.

9. CHRONIC CONDITIONS (E.G., ASTHMA, BRONCHITIS)

Asthma is a chronic lung disease of the lower airways characterized by inflammation, narrowing, and increased production of thick mucous causing plugs. Signs and symptoms include chest tightness, wheezing, cough, accessory muscle use, cyanosis, and respiratory acidosis caused by high levels of CO2.

Acute bronchitis is inflammation of the bronchial tree with partial obstruction, increased secretions, and constriction of the bronchi. This results in abnormally deflated portions of the lung. Localized crackles, expiratory wheezes, tachypnea, cyanosis, a harsh cough, mucoid sputum, fever, and chills characterize acute bronchitis. Complications include pneumonia.

10. FAILURE TO WEAN FROM MECHANICAL VENTILATION

Weaning from mechanical ventilation is an organized process that cannot be initiated until the patient is hemodynamically stable. Arterial blood gases are constantly monitored as well as FiO2 and end-tidal CO2 (ETCO2). Indicators for initiation of weaning include baseline mental status, presence of cough and gag reflexes, absence of fever, spontaneous respiratory effort, normal acid-base balance, oxyhemoglobin ≥ or PaO2 ≥ 60 mm Hg (as long as the patient does not have a cyanotic heart defect), FiO2 < 0.5, PEEP < 7 cm H2O, stable hemodynamics, stable ventilation support ≥ 24 hours, and no planned procedures that will require sedation for the next 12 hours.

11. PULMONARY HYPERTENSION

Pulmonary hypertension is a potentially lethal congenital or acquired condition that is caused by either increased blood flow or increased resistance to blood flow in the pulmonary vasculature. Another definition of pulmonary hypertension is pulmonary artery pressure (PAP) that is greater than one fourth of the systemic pressure. The goal of therapy is to relax the pulmonary vessels and prevent vascular remodeling leading to irreversible pulmonary hypertension. Increased pulmonary blood flow can lead to pulmonary arterial muscle wall thickening and right ventricular strain.

Inhaled nitric oxide is administered for the treatment of pulmonary hypertension. The onset is 1-3 minutes and the half-life is 3-6 seconds. Weaning must be done slowly to avoid worsening increasing pulmonary artery pressure, hypotension, and oxygenation. The desired effect of inhaled nitric oxide is to increase V/Q matching. Methemoglobinemia toxicity is commonly seen with treatment at high doses and for prolonged periods of time, but still requires slow weaning.

12. STATUS ASTHMATICUS

Status asthmaticus is severe exacerbation of asthma characterized by diffuse obstructive disease caused by airway inflammation, mucosal edema, increased mucus production, and bronchospasm. The process begins with submucosal inflammatory infiltrates in the bronchial tree that activates mast cells, epithelial cells, and T lymphocytes that create proinflammatory cytokines. Inflammatory changes lead to epithelial destruction, nerve end exposure, and airway hyper reactivity.

13. THORACIC SURGERY

Bronchoscopy may be performed at bedside in a critical care setting by placing a scope down the patient's nose, mouth, or artificial airway. Bronchoscopes have fiber optic capabilities as well as ventilation ports, suction, and the ability to collect specimens. Complications of bronchoscopy include cardiac arrhythmias, laryngeal edema, pulmonary hemorrhage, laryngospasm, hypoxemia, bronchial tear, pneumothorax, epistaxis, and pulmonary hemorrhage. Patients with chronic lung disease may require more recovery time to return to baseline.

Thoracentesis is a procedure that is performed at bedside to remove fluid or air from the pleural space, such as in treatment of pleural effusion or empyema. Complications include pain, pneumothorax, and re-expansion pulmonary edema. Signs and symptoms of re-expansion pulmonary edema include uncontrollable coughing and shortness of breath, which may occur when a large amount of fluid is removed from the pleural space. Exhibition of these signs and symptoms necessitates stopping the procedure.

14. THORACIC TRAUMA (E.G., FRACTURED RIB, LUNG CONTUSION, TRACHEAL PERFORATION)

Hemothorax is an accumulation of blood in the pleural cavity. Significant hemorrhage and hemothorax are consistent with poor systemic perfusion and respiratory compromise. Rib fractures from thoracic trauma inhibit coughing and deep breathing due to pain. Pain leads to shallow breathing, which could lead to atelectasis and pneumonia. Deep breathing can be performed with an incentive spirometer or by encouraging patients to blow bubbles and use a pinwheel. Patients with rib fractures may find using a towel, blanket, or stuffed animal to splint the ribs and reduce pain when coughing.

Pulmonary contusions are bruises in the lung that manifest as hemorrhage, followed by alveolar and interstitial edema. Edema may remain localized, or it may spread. Edema affects the capillaries, causing decreased compliance, increased pulmonary vascular resistance, and decreased blood flow resulting in ventilation-perfusion mismatch. Positioning the patient with the injured side up maximizes ventilation and perfusion.

Chapter 3

I. Clinical Judgment:
C.
Endocrine/Hematology/Gastrointestinal/ Renal/Integumentary (19%) = 28.5 questions

1. ENDOCRINE
A. ACUTE HYPOGLYCEMIA

Acute hypoglycemia is defined as serum glucose less than 50 mg/dL. Lack of glucose leads to lack of energy, cell death (especially in the brain), and metabolism of fat for energy (ketotic hypoglycemia). Complications of acute hypoglycemia include neuronal death, coma, seizures, neurological deficits, and death.

B. DIABETES INSIPIDUS

Diabetes insipidus (DI) is characterized by large amounts of urine output due to low levels of antidiuretic (ADH), thus it necessitates fluid replacement to prevent dehydration. Intake, output, and electrolytes must be monitored vigilantly. Vasopressin intravenous (IV) or subcutaneously (SQ) and desmopressin (DDAVP) 5-20 mcg intranasally every 24 hours are used in the treatment of diabetes insipidus (DI) to replace antidiuretic hormone (ADH), increase water reabsorption in the nephron, and prevent as well as control polydipsia and polyuria.

10. A patient with diabetes insipidus exhibits polyuria. The *most likely* reason is
a. High serum blood glucose levels
b. Low antidiuretic hormone levels
c. High urine osmolality
d. Low serum sodium levels

(See Chapter 7 for answers)

C. DIABETIC KETOACIDOSIS

Diabetic ketoacidosis (DKA) is a life-threatening complication of diabetes mellitus characterized by hyperglycemia, ketoacidosis, hyperosmolality, volume depletion, and acidosis. Hypovolemia must be corrected rapidly to prevent hypovolemic shock. Cerebral edema is a rare but potentially fatal complication of DKA.

D. HYPERGLYCEMIA

Hyperglycemia promotes osmotic diuresis, producing polyuria, polydipsia, and cellular and intravascular fluid depletion. The breakdown of body fat leads to the release of excessive ketones, which produces metabolic acidosis.

E. INBORN ERRORS OF METABOLISM

Inborn errors of metabolism include maple sugar urine disease, which is an inability to break down the amino acids leucine, isoleucine, and valine. Symptoms include lethargy, sweet smelling urine, feeding difficulties, and vomiting.

F. SYNDROME OF INAPPROPRIATE SECRETION OF ANTIDIURETIC HORMONE (SIADH)

Syndrome of inappropriate antidiuretic hormone (SIADH) is characterized by excessive amounts of ADH resulting in water retention. Hyponatremia is a result of hemodilution. Conditions associated with SIADH include meningitis, head trauma, cerebral tumors, cerebral hemorrhage, pulmonary disease, chronically ill or malnourished children, and spinal surgery. The first symptom is low urine output in the absence of hypovolemia.

2. HEMATOLOGY/IMMUNOLOGY
A. ANEMIA

Anemia is defined as low hemoglobin and hematocrit. Signs and symptoms of anemia vary depending on severity, and some patients may be asymptomatic. Anemia leads to tachypnea, tachycardia, hypotension, oliguria, and hyperglycemia due to a compensatory response caused by decreased oxygen delivery. Causes of anemia include blood loss, decreased production, splenic sequestration, and hemolysis.

B. COAGULOPATHIES (E.G., ITP, DIC, HIT)

Immune thrombocytopenic purpura (ITP) is classified by normal PTT (25-40 seconds), normal PT (12-15 seconds), decreased platelets (<150,000/mm3), and normal fibrin split products (FSP) levels. Platelets are decreased due to an immune-mediation. The exact cause is unknown, but ITP typically follows a viral infections. Antibodies are developed against platelets leading to platelet destruction, which leads to bleeding into the skin.

Disseminated intravascular coagulation (DIC) is an abnormal coagulation process causing accelerated normal clotting, a decrease in clotting factors and platelets, and uncontrolled bleeding. Platelets are decreased, PT/PTT are prolonged, fibrinogen is decreased, FSP is elevated, and D-dimer is elevated.

Heparin-induced thrombocytopenia (HIT) is classified by unexplained 50% or greater reduction in platelet count after 5 or more days of heparin therapy. An antibody-antigen reaction on the surface of platelets leads to creation of microparticles made of platelets. The microparticles signal the clotting cascade, which produces thromboemboli.

C. IMMUNE DEFICIENCIES

Immunodeficiency is a permanent state of decreased function of the immune system while immunosuppression is a temporary impairment. Immunocompromise is the result of both immunodeficiency and immunosuppression.

D. LEUKOPENIA

Leukopenia is defined as low white blood cell count (WBC). Evaluation of the patient's absolute neutrophil count (ANC) is a better indicator of the patient's ability to fight infection than evaluation of WBC. Patients are considered neutropenic with an ANC $1000/mm^3$ in infants less than 1 year old and $1500/mm^3$ in children older than 1 year. Severe neutropenia is demonstrated with an ANC less than $500/mm^3$.

E. ONCOLOGIC COMPLICATIONS

Tumor lysis syndrome (TLS) is an oncologic complication that can lead to acute renal failure (ARF). It usually occurs after effective chemotherapy or radiation therapy, but it can also occur after treatment with glucocorticoids, antiestrogen tamoxifen, and interferon. TLS leads to rapid release of intracellular metabolites that exceeds the capability of the kidneys to excrete. Potential effects include hyperuricemia, hypocalcemia, hyperphosphatemia, hyperkalemia, and hyperxanthinemia. Treatment of TLS is prevention with vigorous hydration and allopurinol before cancer treatment.

Hyperleukocytosis is defined as increased white blood cell count, greater than 100,000/mm^3. White blood cells may clump as a result of increased blood viscosity leading to obstruction of blood vessels and development of thrombi in the microcirculation.

11. A patient with acute lymphoblastic leukemia (ALL) is on a norepinephrine drip for septic shock after induction chemotherapy 2 days prior. The last set of laboratory findings are as follows:

Potassium	5.9 mEq/L
Phosphorus	4.9 mg/dL
Calcium	7.8 mg/dL
BUN	7.5 mmol/L

The nurse anticipates which of the following interventions?
a. Vigorous IV hydration
b. Increasing the norepinephrine drip
c. Administration of Kayexalate
d. Administration of IV calcium chloride

F. SICKLE CELL CRISIS

Sickle cell disease describes a genetic mutation, which leads to crescent or sickle shaped red blood cells when oxygen saturations fall. Vasoocclusive crises may involve the central nervous system (CNS), bone, lungs, or other visceral organs. Sickled cells clump causing splenic sequestration, cerebrovascular accident (CVA), acute chest syndrome, and priapism. Complications include cholelithiasis, jaundice, slowed growth, stroke, and gallstones. Splenic sequestration crisis is seen in young children and results in trapping of red blood cells (RBCs) in the spleen with subsequent anemia, hypotension, splenomegaly (which is easily palpated), and shock. The cause of splenic sequestration is unknown.

12. Sickle cell disease is suspected in an 8-year-old. Diagnostic findings consistent with this diagnosis include
a. Abnormal peripheral blood smear and anemia
b. Positive blood cultures and hyperglycemia
c. Elevated aspartate aminotransferase (AST) and alanine aminotransferase (ALT)
d. Leukocytosis and bandemia

G. THROMBOCYTOPENIA

Thrombocytopenia is defined as lower than normal amount of platelets circulating in the blood. The most common causes include decreased production of platelets, and sequestration of platelets. Normal platelet count is 150,000-400,000/mm^3 and severe thrombocytopenia is less than 20,000/mm^3.

3. GASTROINTESTINAL
A. ACUTE ABDOMINAL TRAUMA

Cullen's sign is described as edema and bruising at the umbilicus and may be seen after abdominal trauma due to bleeding into the subcutaneous tissues. Turner's may be seen after abdominal trauma and is described as bruising over the flank. Splenic laceration is characterized by referred pain to the left shoulder due to compression of the left upper quadrant of the abdomen, also known as a positive Kehr's sign. Renal trauma is typically characterized by hematuria. Liver laceration is consistent with abdominal pain, guarding, and right upper quadrant abdominal tenderness.

Intra-abdominal pressure monitoring is a method of measuring pressure in the abdomen and assess for abdominal compartment syndrome. Normal intra-abdominal pressures (IAP) are 0-12 mmHg. Intra-abdominal pressures are measured using a foley with a transducer. Grade 1 intra-abdominal hypertension (IAH) is defined as a sustained pressure of 12-15 mmHg. Grade II IAH is 16-10 mmHg. Grade III IAH is 21-15 mmHg. Grade IV is > 25 mmHg. Abdominal compartment syndrome (ACS) is defined as sustained pressures > 20 mmHg. Risk factors for IAH/ACS include decreased abdominal wall compliance, increased intra-luminal contents, increased abdominal contents, and capillary leak (as seen in fluid resuscitation).

B. ACUTE GI HEMORRHAGE

Acute GI hemorrhage requires rapid response by the critical care team, especially if severe hemorrhage is present. The nurse can anticipate administration of fresh frozen plasma, packed red blood cells, platelets, and Vitamin K to stop clinical evidence of bleeding.

13. Octreotide may be used in the treatment of which patient?
a. Rotavirus infection
b. Hyperbilirubinemia
c. Hemorrhagic pancreatitis
d. Ascites

C. BOWEL INFARCTION/OBSTRUCTION/ PERFORATION (E.G., MESENTERIC ISCHEMIA, ADHESIONS)

The mesenteric artery delivers blood from the aorta to the GI tract. Narrowing or blocking of the mesenteric artery causes mesenteric ischemia. Ischemia may also be caused by a blood clot blocking the artery. Blood tinged stool, if present, indicates that the bowel may be becoming gangrenous. The patient must be stabilized with fluid resuscitation and adequate ventilation before emergent surgery.

D. GASTROESOPHAGEAL REFLUX

Gastroesophageal reflux is defined as stomach contents back into the esophagus. Reflux may be silent, or it may cause pain, discomfort, neck arching, coughing, swallowing, or emesis. Presence of a nasogastric (NG) or nasoduodenal (ND) tube may contribute to reflux as the rube may prevent closure of the gastroesophageal sphincter.

E. GI ABNORMALITIES (E.G., OMPHALOCELE, GASTROSCHISIS, VOLVULUS, IMPERFORATE ANUS, HIRSCHSPRUNG DISEASE, MALROTATION, INTUSSUSCEPTION)

Congenital gastrointestinal (GI) abnormalities are best managed if they are diagnosed prenatally in order to allow for a birth plan that includes treatment at a tertiary care facility for surgical intervention. Early enteral feeding, and prevention or treatment of postoperative complications are also vital. Failure to pass meconium in the first 24 hours of life is a strong indicator of a congenital GI abnormality.

F. GI SURGERIES

Perforation is a complication of EGD or any invasive GI procedure. Inadvertent tears can occur in the esophagus, stomach, or duodenum. Assessment findings include tachycardia, hypotension, low central venous pressure (CVP), pain, fever, vomiting, tachypnea, and difficulty swallowing. Other complications include infection and bleeding from the biopsy site.

G. HEPATIC FAILURE/COMA (E.G., PORTAL HYPERTENSION, CIRRHOSIS, ESOPHAGEAL VARICES, FULMINANT HEPATITIS, BILIARY ATRESIA)

Causes of hepatic failure include portal-systemic shunting, fulminant liver failure, neurologic pathophysiology (which is unclear), renal pathophysiology, and hematologic pathophysiology (including coagulopathy and hypersplenism). Liver damage and scarring are causes of cirrhosis. Outflow obstruction of the liver into the inferior vena cava (IVC) causes portal hypertension and esophageal varices.

Treatment for esophageal varices includes initiation of a Vasopressin drip, initiation of an Octreotide drip, endoscopic scleropathy, band ligation, and surgical placement of a Sengstaken-Blakemore tube. Liver transplant and the Kasai procedure are surgical interventions for biliary atresia. Heparin therapy is contraindicated in treating esophageal varices due to increased risk for more bleeding.

Biliary atresia is a congenital condition involving the absence of biliary ducts inside or outside of the liver (intrahepatic or extrahepatic). Bile flow becomes obstructed causing fibrosis and cirrhosis. Surgical intervention with the Kasai procedure or a liver transplant is necessary in children with biliary atresia to restore bile flow.

14. A child develops tachycardia on postop day 5 after abdominal surgery. The nurse's next action is to

a. Perform pulmonary hygiene

b. Administer rectal acetaminophen

c. Inspect the abdominal incision

d. Assess bilateral lung sounds

H. MALNUTRITION AND MALABSORPTION

Malnutrition and malabsorption may be treated with a NG or ND tube. Aspirating and refeeding residual volume is controversial in pediatrics. Residual volumes should be measured and recorded according to the policy of the facility. Signs of feeding intolerance include vomiting, diarrhea, and abdominal distension.

4. RENAL/GENITOURINARY
A. *ACUTE KIDNEY INJURY (AKI), ACUTE RENAL FAILURE, ACUTE TUBULAR NECROSIS (ATN)*

Acute renal failure is a sudden decrease in kidney function leading to increased buildup of nitrogenous waste products in the blood such as products of protein metabolism, urea, and creatinine. Injury to the distal tubules impairs the ability of the kidneys to excrete potassium and creatinine, causing hyperkalemia, increased creatinine levels, and increased blood urea nitrogen (BUN). Oliguria is typically present, but not always as polyuria may be seen with acute kidney injury. Acute renal injury may be caused by hypovolemia, hypotension, shock, renal artery thrombosis, or aortic thrombosis.

B. *CHRONIC KIDNEY DISEASE*

Chronic kidney disease (CKD) may result from malformation of the renal system, infection, genetic renal disorders, trauma, or glomerular disease. Symptoms may seem vague. They include fatigue, anorexia, nausea, abdominal pain, growth failure, polyuria, polydipsia, edema (especially around the eyes), oliguria, pallor, skin rashes, arthritis, and a history of a previous renal or urologic disease. Pathophysiology includes uremia, sodium and water retention, hyperkalemia, acidosis, hypocalcemia, hyperphosphatemia, anemia, uremic encephalopathy, and neuropathy. Hypertension is managed with diuretics.

15. The nurse is admitting a child with chronic kidney disease (CKD). The nurse should assess which of the following *first*?
a.   Sodium level
b.   Blood glucose level
c.   Blood urea nitrogen (BUN)
d.   Hemoglobin level

C. INFECTIONS

Patients are at great risk for infection after renal transplant because patients are immunocompromised and steroids are rapidly weaned. Patients are especially at risk if an augmented bladder or complete diversion of urine is present. Urinary catheters must be secured with no tension and drainage bags must be below the level of the bladder. Incisions must be closely monitored days after transplant for edema, redness, and/or purulent drainage. Strict hand washing is vital for everyone who comes in contact with the patient. The child's temperature and WBC should be monitored and signs of infections should be reported to the licensed independent practitioner (LIP) immediately for blood/urine cultures and administration of antibiotics.

D. LIFE-THREATENING ELECTROLYTE IMBALANCES

Osmolality refers to the concentration of solutes (electrolytes and proteins) per liter of fluid. Sodium is the primary electrolyte affecting serum osmolality. An acute fall in sodium may result in an intracellular water shift leading to cerebral edema.

	Normal	DI	SIADH
Serum Na	135-145 mEq/L	↑	↓
Urine Na	60-100 mEq/L	↓	↑
Serum osmolality	275-300 mOsm/kg	↑	↓
Urine osmolality	300-800 mOsm/kg	↓	↑
Urine spec grav	1.005-1.020	↓	↑
Urine output	1-2 mL/kg/hr	↑	↓

Serum potassium concentration and pH have an inverse relationship in response to potassium and hydrogen ions shifting in a reciprocal manner into and out of the cell. Hormones affecting fluid and electrolyte balance include ADH, aldosterone, and natriuretic peptides.

16. The nurse is caring for a child with acute renal failure. The nurse expects which of the following assessment findings?
a.   Hypernatremia
b.   Hypercalcemia
c.   Hyperkalemia
d.   Hypophosphatemia

5. INTEGUMENTARY
A. IV INFILTRATION

IV infiltration is a spectrum from mild to severe. Severe IV infiltration may develop into compartment syndrome. Compartment syndrome occurs when pressure in the myofascial compartment is greater than capillary perfusion pressure, leading to decreased blood flow to the tissues within. Risk factors for include hemorrhage, edema, extravasation, extreme muscle inactivity, and presence of equipment (dressings, casts).

Most fractures are simple and nondisplaced, requiring only casting. While swelling of the fingers and toes as well as odor from the cast are part of the assessment, sharp pain, numbness, tenseness, paresthesia, decreased sensation, and no sensation may indicate compartment syndrome. Elevating the extremity to the level of the heart may relieve slight swelling of the fingers.

B. PRESSURE ULCER

Frequent turning and progressive mobility are vital in critically ill children. Children with pressure ulcers on the sacrum or coccyx who have diarrhea require vigilant perineal care.

C. WOUNDS
I. INFECTIOUS
II. SURGICAL
III. TRAUMA

Care of infectious wounds may include use of a vacuum-assisted closure (VAC). Vigilant assessment is required to ensure that the device is functioning properly.

Scald and burn marks must be reviewed for abuse or neglect. Children with severe burns should be transferred to a burn center.

17. A child receiving negative pressure wound therapy (NPWT) to a deep sternal wound infection after cardiac surgery has saturated the foam dressing and filled the drainage container 3 hours after the dressing was changed. The *first* intervention by the nurse is to
a. Notify the licensed independent practitioner (LIP)
b. Replace it with a wet to dry sterile dressing
c. Contact the wound ostomy continence nurse (WOCN)
d. Quantify and document the amount of blood loss

Stephanie Doig

Chapter 4

I. Clinical Judgment: D. Musculoskeletal/ Neurology/Psychosocial (16%) = 24 questions

1. MUSCULOSKELETAL
A. INFECTIONS

Osteomyelitis is an infection of the bone. In children, the long bones are most often affected, meaning the arms and legs. Pain, fever, and swelling at the affected site may be noted.

2. NEUROLOGY
A.   ACUTE SPINAL CORD INJURY

Spinal cord injury may be complete or incomplete, which correlates with complete or partial loss of sensory and motor function below the level of injury. Nursing diagnoses include altered respiratory function (if the injury is high on the cervical spine), altered cardiac output related to autonomic nervous system dysfunction, potential for impaired gas exchange related to pulmonary emboli from immobility, potential for alteration in skin integrity, potential for pulmonary infection related to artificial airway, alteration in temperature regulation related to damage to central thermoregulatory centers, and altered elimination patterns related to decreased innervation of viscera.

B. BRAIN DEATH

Most states have determined that brain death guidelines for infants, children, and adults include one or two of the following conditions: 1. irreversible cessation of breathing and circulation OR 2. irreversible cessation of whole-brain functions (such as cortical or brainstem). The process in confirming brain death may vary from state to state. Presence of doll's eyes and absence of a nystagmus with cold calorics indicates absence of oculocephalic and oculovestibular reflexes.

A normal oculovestibular reflex is seen when cold water is flushed into the ears causing nystagmus. Absence of this reflex is abnormal and may indicate brain death. A normal oculocephalic reflex is present when the head is rapidly turned to one side and the eyes deviate to the opposite side of head movement. Presence of doll's eyes may be indicative of brain death. The time allowed following disconnection from the ventilator to allow PaCO2 to increase in order to stimulate a spontaneous breath is 5-10 minutes.

18. A 3-week-old is awaiting brain death testing. The mother tells the nurse she is sure the baby cannot be brain dead because she sees the baby's feet move when she touches the leg. The nurse's best response is

a. "These movements are likely spinal cord reflexes, which are reflexes of the spinal cord that run from the feet to the spinal cord and back."

b. "Your baby still has spinal cord reflexes, which may continue despite cerebral cortex injury and brain death."

c. "We will have to wait to see the results of the brain death testing to determine from where the movement is being generated."

d. "The movement that you're seeing is not considered purposeful movement, such as tracking with the eyes, sucking, or grasping an object."

C. *CONGENITAL NEUROLOGICAL ABNORMALITIES (E.G., AV MALFORMATION, MYELOMENINGOCELE, ENCEPHALOCELE)*

Arteriovenous malformation (AVM) is an abnormal connection between the arteries and veins in the brain, making it the most common cause of intracranial hemorrhage in children. Treatment options include surgery, radiosurgery, and irradiation depending on the patient's condition. Dilated pupils and nystagmus are not symptoms of AVM. Seizures are seen if the AVM has hemorrhaged.

AVM places patients at risk for hemorrhage and rebleeding after surgery. Signs and symptoms of hemorrhage include severe headache, seizures, decreased level of consciousness, hypotonia, irritability, decreased hemoglobin, and abnormal eye movements in a patient that is slowly deteriorating. Signs and symptoms in a rapidly deteriorating patient include coma, apnea, seizures, and unreactive pupils. Creating a calm environment keeps intracranial pressure (ICP) low and decreases vasospasm.

The cause of congenital neurologic abnormalities is unknown. A ventriculoperitoneal shunt may be indicated if hydrocephalus is present in order to decrease intracranial pressures. Nursing diagnoses include potential for infection after surgery, potential for decreased cardiac output related to anaphylactic shock from latex hypersensitivity, altered cerebral tissue perfusion related to increased ICP due to hydrocephalus, and altered elimination related to decreased innervation of bladder, urinary sphincter, and lower intestines.

D.   ENCEPHALOPATHY

Hepatic encephalopathy is the leading cause of morbidity and mortality in patients with liver failure. Several theories exist, but the etiology is unknown. Hepatic encephalopathy leads to cerebral edema that is associated with astrocyte swelling and increased brain water content causing increased intracranial pressure. Jaundice is yellowing of the skin. Esophageal varices are distended veins in the esophagus from increased due to obstruction of blood flow to the liver. Asterixis is hand flapping, which is a myoclonic jerking of the hands that may be seen in chronic liver failure.

Increased ICP leads to compression of the oculomotor nerve resulting in pupil dilation, decreased pupil constriction, or absent pupil constriction. Irritability followed by lethargy is a sign of increased ICP. Patients with increased ICP may exhibit a decrease in purposeful movement, flaccidity, and/or posturing. Bradycardia is a late sign of increased ICP.

Mannitol is an osmotic agent used for the treatment of intracranial hypertension through osmotic and vasoactive actions. Water shifts from the intracellular space to the extracellular space and decreases blood viscosity leading to an increase in cerebral blood flow and an increase in oxygenation to tissues. The rapid fluid shift leads to a decrease in ICP.

E. HEAD TRAUMA

Head injuries are typically the result of blunt force from motor-vehicle accidents, bicycle accidents, falls, and child abuse. Head injuries range from mild to severe in severity, depending on presentation and Glascow Coma Scale. Goals of treatment include promoting oxygenation and ventilation, maintaining normal PCO2 levels, maintaining normal ICP levels, maximizing ventricular drainage of CSF, administration of diuretics (including mannitol and lasix), maximizing venous drainage by keeping the head of bed elevated, maximizing cerebral perfusion pressure (CPP) and systemic arterial pressure with temperature and seizure control, and maintaining normothermia with consideration of hypothermia. Hyperthermia should be avoided.

F. HEMORRHAGE
I. INTRACRANIAL (ICH)
II. INTRAVENTRICULAR (IVH)
III. SUBARACHNOID (TRAUMATIC OR ANEURYSMAL)

Intracranial hemorrhage is the result of thrombocytopenia or an AVM with increased intracranial pressure that has spontaneously ruptured. Signs and symptoms include rapid deterioration, seizures, headaches, poor appetite, vomiting, vision changes, ataxia, slurred speech, and reports of weakness or numbness.

A subdural hematoma is a collection of blood in between the dura and the brain. Symptoms include disorientation, headache, loss of consciousness, seizures, slurred speech, weakness, nausea, and vomiting. Patient care should be clustered in order to allow for adequate rest periods because nursing care is known to directly increase intracranial pressure.

19. A school-aged child recovering from arteriovenous (AV) malformation repair begins to experience emesis, headache, and altered mental status. The *most likely* cause is
a. Brainstem herniation
b. Encephalopathy
c. Cerebrovascular accident
d. Diabetes insipidus

(See Chapter 7 for answers)

G. HYDROCEPHALUS

Hydrocephalus may be congenital or acquired in etiology. Acquired hydrocephalus is the result of obstructive lesions such as neoplasms, hemorrhage, infections, and trauma. Older children present differently than infants, with signs and symptoms of headache, nausea, vomiting, headache, unsteady gait, history of falling, deterioration in school performance, urinary incontinence, papilledema (swelling of the optic disc), diplopia (double vision), seizures, and behavioral changes such as irritability, fatigue, and personality changes.

Poor feeding and a high-pitched cry are indicative of hydrocephalus and increased intracranial pressure. The nurse should anticipate preparation for a lumbar puncture for cerebrospinal (CSF) analysis. Other signs and symptoms of hydrocephalus in an infant include increased head circumference, setting-sun sign (sclera that are visible above the iris), bulging fontanelles, protruding scalp veins, and thin, shiny skin on the scalp.

The Cushing reflex, or the Cushing triad, is seen in as a late sign of significantly increased ICP. It is an ominous sign and may occur with cerebral brainstem herniation. Another late sign of increased ICP is hypotension. Other assessment findings may include decorticate posturing (abnormal and rigid flexion of the arms and legs), decerebrate posturing (abnormal and rigid extension of the arms and legs), unequal pupil size, and decreased pupil reaction to light.

H. ISCHEMIC STROKE

Ischemic stroke is the result of interruption of blood flow from a thrombotic or embolic event. Pediatric patients at risk include sickle cell disease, protein C disorders, polycythemia, anemia, and prolonged vasoconstriction. Signs and symptoms include hemiparesis, unilateral headache, dizziness, fatigue, aphasia, seizures, and signs and symptoms of hydrocephalus.

Heparin therapy is standard treatment for ischemic stroke in children. Treatment with tissue plasminogen activator (tPA) is standard care in adults, but is not FDA approved in children. After the patient has imaging confirming no hemorrhage, Heparin therapy is initiated with a bolus of 75 units/kg and an infusion rate of 15 units/kg/hr. Coags are drawn 1 hour after infusion initiation and the dose is adjusted to obtain a target aPTT of 60-85 seconds.

I. NEUROLOGIC INFECTIOUS DISEASE (E.G., VIRAL, BACTERIAL, FUNGAL)

Meningitis is inflammation of the meninges that may be bacterial or viral in nature. Petechial rash is associated with *Neisseria meningitidis*. *N. meningitidis* is the most common cause of bacterial meningitis in children over 2 months old. Group B streptococcus is associated with neonates, while mycobacterium tuberculosis is uncommon in the United States. Cryptococcal meningitis is most often found in patients with weakened immune systems.

A positive Brudzinski sign, involuntary flexion of the hips and knees with passive neck flexion, is indicative of bacterial meningitis. Other signs and symptoms of bacterial meningitis include nuchal rigidity (neck stiffness), Kernig's sign (back pain and resistance with passive extension of lower legs), fever, emesis, headache, and altered level of consciousness. Signs and symptoms of viral meningitis are similar, but typically have a more mild clinical presentation.

CSF findings for bacterial meningitis includes increased WBC count, increased protein (greater than 30 mg/dL), decreased glucose (less than 40 mg/dL), positive Gram stain, positive cultures for organism, and turbid or cloudy color. Computed tomography (CT) and magnetic resonance imaging (MRI) results may be abnormal, but these images do not predict prognosis or the degree of encephalitis.

Viral meningitis is less common than bacterial meningitis. The pathological process of viral meningitis is unclear, but it may enter and colonize the body via the nasopharynx and spread to the blood and then the CNS. The clinical course is typically self-limiting, lasting 7-14 days. CSF culture for bacteria is negative. The most common pathogens of viral meningitis include enteroviruses, mumps, herpes simplex type 1, adenoviruses, and California virus.

J. NEUROMUSCULAR DISORDERS

Guillan-Barre Syndrome (GBS) is a reversible, rapidly progressive autoimmune response affecting the motor and sensory pathways of the peripheral nervous system and autonomic function of cranial nerves, which leads to paralysis and possible respiratory failure. Symptoms progress over a period of hours to days. Symptoms include weakness, paresthesias, sensory changes, cranial nerve dysfunction, and autonomic dysfunction. Continuous monitoring is necessary in order to intervene and prevent complications of respiratory arrest such as atelectasis, pneumonia, and pneumothorax. Autonomic dysfunction may produce hypertension and tachycardia requiring intervention with beta-blockers.

K. NEUROSURGERY

Postoperative care of a patient immediately after neurosurgery includes assessing the airway, oxygenation, ventilation, systemic perfusion, and neurological status. The patient is positioned with the head of bed elevated to 30 degrees to promote chest expansion, with the head, neck, and body midline. Flexion and hyperextension of the neck must be avoided.

L. SEIZURE DISORDERS

Status epilepticus is a prolonged seizure, lasting 30 minutes or more. The goal of treatment is to reduce the frequency of seizures. Patients leave the hospital on seizure medications such as Keppra, Depakote, Tegretol, and Dilantin. Families must be taught how and when to administer rectal diazepam in case the patient has a seizure lasting greater than 5 minutes outside of the hospital setting.

Febrile seizures are common in young children. High fevers lower the seizure threshold, so the cause is not CNS related. Children typically grow out of febrile seizures by age 5 or 6. Alternating antipyretics to prevent high spikes should control fevers. Pediatric dosing for acetaminophen is 10-15 mg/kg/dose PO/PR every 4-6 hours and dosing for ibuprofen is 4-10 mg/kg/dose PO every 6-8 hours. Children admitted for febrile seizures may receive an electroencephalogram (EEG), but video EEG is not indicated.

M. SPACE OCCUPYING LESIONS (E.G., BRAIN TUMORS)

Space-occupying lesions and tumors are a cause of increased ICP that have unknown etiology. Symptoms are different depending on age of the child, location, and rate of growth. Treatment options include surgery, radiation, and chemotherapy. Close neurological assessment is required in order to monitor ICP, cerebral perfusion pressure (CPP), and any possible side effects of chemotherapy. If surgery is performed, cerebral swelling may be at its peak on postoperative day 3. Steroid therapy may be used for localized edema around the tumor.

N. SPINAL FUSION

Spinal fusion is a surgery performed on spinal cord injury patients to fuse together the vertebrae, providing spinal column support and stability. SIADH and postoperative hemorrhage are not typical complications of spinal fusion. Complications may include cardiovascular defects (such as hypotension, temperature regulation dysfunction, and deep venous thrombosis also known as DVT), pulmonary complications (such as ineffective airway clearance and hypoventilation), risk for contractures, risk for pressure ulcers, and dysfunction of the bowel and bladder.

O. TRAUMATIC BRAIN INJURY (E.G., EPIDURAL, SUBDURAL, CONCUSSION, NON-ACCIDENTAL TRAUMA)

The pathophysiology of traumatic brain injury is divided into primary and secondary injury. Primary injury is the result of the initial trauma, such as hemorrhage, contusion, laceration, and shearing injury. Secondary injury is the body's response to the primary injury, which may cause loss of brain tissue that was not damaged during the initial injury. The biochemical and cellular response of the secondary injury includes tissue ischemia, hypotension, hypercapnia, and brain edema. Hypercapnia causes cerebral vasodilation, increased blood volume, and increased ICP.

Treatment of patients with traumatic brain injury (TBI) includes passing the suction catheter for less than 10 seconds, passing the suction catheter only twice per incident, and hyperoxygenating the patient before and after suctioning the patient. These interventions minimize stimulation of the airway, maintaining low ICP and maximizing CPP. Following cardiac markers is indicated in chest trauma, but not TBI. Initiation of hypothermia protocol and administration of antiarrhythmics are not indicated in TBI.

3. BEHAVIORAL/PSYCHOSOCIAL
A. ABUSE, MALTREATMENT, NEGLECT

Child maltreatment is defined as an act, or failure of a parent or caregiver to act in response to a child's needs, resulting in physical or emotional harm to the child. Health care providers must assess family members of trauma patients in order to ensure that the history provided matches the injuries of the child. Multiples injuries in different stages of healing require further investigation. A patient who does not oppose painful procedures should raise suspicion of child abuse or maltreatment.

B. AGITATION

Identifying agitation and delirium in children is vital and requires fine tuned assessment skills. Causes of agitation and delirium are metabolic, intracranial, endocrine, organ failure, respiratory, and medication-related. Agitation in children may be indicative of pain, which can lead to sleep disturbances, anxiety, nausea, anorexia, and fatigue. Parents and caregivers who know the child best are valuable in the assessment and treatment.

C. DEVELOPMENTAL DELAYS

Patients who have had an anoxic birth injury had a large variety of developmental delays. Further assessment is required in order to know if the patient has the capacity to understand and react to commands such as blinking and moving. The best way to assess pain in developmentally delayed children is to know what the heart rate and blood pressure are when the patient is quietly resting. These values will often increase before the patient begins to wake up.

D. FAILURE TO THRIVE

Failure to thrive is defined as caloric intake that is insufficient to meet the needs of the body, thus compromising growth. Failure to thrive is often the first sign of congenital heart disease in infants.

E. MEDICAL NON-ADHERENCE

Medical non-adherence may occur due to many reasons such as lack of financial resources, decreased understanding of disease processes, and psychological disorders (anxiety, depression, etc.). Identifying barriers is the first step in changing behavior. Nurses are in the best position to learn barriers because they spend the most time at the bedside.

F. SUICIDAL IDEATION AND/OR BEHAVIORS

The goal of supporting the family of a child who has attempted suicide is to promote the family's values, interests, and goals. The best way to support the patient's and family's needs are to listen to the concerns, feelings, and questions of all family members while enlisting support of other resources, such as social work or spiritual resources, as necessary. The family's values should be accepted in a nonjudgmental manner.

Stephanie Doig

Chapter 5

I. Clinical Judgment: E. Multisystem (14%) = 21 questions

1. ASPHYXIA

Acute asphyxia is an inhalation injury often seen in burn patients as a result of carbon monoxide poisoning. The most common sources of carbon monoxide poisoning are motor vehicle exhaust, smoke from fires, engine fumes, and non-electric heaters. Airway injury is caused by the chemical inhalation of the by-products of combustion. Cerebral hypoxemia from smoke leads to neurological dysfunction in the form of confusion.

Carbon monoxide poisoning is an inhalation injury that can cause acute asphyxia. House fires, exhaust from automobiles, gas-powered equipment (furnaces, space heaters, ovens, hot water heaters), and wood- and coal-burning stoves and fireplaces can lead to toxicity of the tasteless, odorless gas. Symptoms include headache, nausea, and lethargy, which are all related to hypoxemia. Cerebral hypoxia can lead to cerebral edema with lasting neurologic effects if damage is severe. Tachypnea and cyanosis may be absent because the body's peripheral chemoreceptors perceive normal partial pressure of oxygen in arterial blood (PaO2). Upper airway edema and facial edema are expected with carbon monoxide caused by smoke inhalation.

2. COMORBIDITY IN PATIENTS WITH TRANSPLANT HISTORY

Post transplant lymphoproliferative disease (PTLD) is common in renal transplant patients undergoing immunosuppressive therapy. It is the development of continually proliferating lymphocytes (typically B lymphocytes), which is stimulated by a virus such as Eppstein-Barr Virus (EBV). EBV (which is the most common virus to stimulate proliferation), cytomegalovirus (CMV), herpes simplex virus (HSV), BK virus, varicella, and pneumocystis carinii pneumonia (PCP).

3. END OF LIFE

Parents bear the primary responsibility for filtering information from the healthcare team to the child. Open communication, using open-ended questions, is recommended in life-threatening or life-limiting circumstances. Word choice is extremely important for healthcare providers caring for terminally ill children.

Organ donation is likely to be a sensitive subject for a family who is losing a member. Most local organ donation teams prefer that their coordinators approach the family and provide education, as they have been specifically trained for the task. If it is determined that a child may be a candidate for donation, the role of the nurse is to follow the lead of the donation team. The nurse may be asked to provide a private area for the family to meet.

4. HEALTHCARE-ASSOCIATED INFECTIONS (HAI)

A. CENTRAL LINE-ASSOCIATED BLOODSTREAM INFECTIONS (CLABSI)

Use of chlorhexidine for antisepsis is not recommended in children under 2 months old. Sterile technique is required when changing central venous catheter (CVC) dressings. Ensuring proper hand hygiene after changing the dressing is extremely important after gloves have been removed. Daily review of line necessity and prompt removal of unnecessary lines are practices that have been shown to reduce the incidence of central line-associated bloodstream infections. Use of maximal barrier precautions includes use of a cap, mask, sterile gown, sterile gloves, and sterile drape. Supplies should be kept in a central line cart that is easily accessible.

B. CATHETER-ASSOCIATED URINARY TRACT INFECTION (CAUTI)

Most critically ill children require a urinary drainage catheter in order to measure urine accurately. The drainage bag should be kept below the level of the bladder to prevent urine backflow and maintain unobstructed flow of urine. The need for urinary drainage catheters should be reviewed daily for necessity and should the catheter should be removed as soon as possible. Routine, scheduled replacement of urinary catheters is not recommended.

C. VAP (I.E., VENTILATOR-ASSOCIATED EVENT OR VAE)

Ventilator-associated pneumonia (VAP) is a hospital-acquired infection that was not present before mechanical ventilation and occurs more than 48 hours after initiation of mechanical ventilation. Risk factors for pediatrics include altered mental status, immunodeficiency, prolonged mechanical ventilation, neuromuscular blockade, primary bloodstream infection, severe traumatic brain injury, burn injury, steroids, reintubation, and congenital neuromuscular weakness.

5. HEMOLYTIC UREMIC SYNDROME (HUS)

HUS is a thrombotic microangiopathic disease involving endothelial damage leading to platelet and fibrin deposits in small vessels. It is characterized by acute hemolytic anemia, thrombocytopenia, and acute kidney injury (AKI). Nursing management includes recognition and treatment of neurologic complications, fluid and electrolyte assessment, administration of packed red blood cells (PRBCs), and management of hypertension

6. HYPOTENSION

Aggressive fluid resuscitation with normal saline leads to hypokalemia, hypernatremia, and metabolic acidosis due to dilution of the blood. Metabolic acidosis results from hyperchloremia, an increase in chloride ions, excretion of bicarbonate by the kidneys, and a decrease in pH.

7. INFECTIOUS DISEASES

A. MULTIDRUG-RESISTANT ORGANISMS (E.G., MRSA, VRE, CRE)

Multidrug resistant infectious diseases, such as Methicillin-resistant Staphylococcus aureus (MRSA) and Vancomycin-resistant enterococcus (VRE), as well as contagious conditions like influenza, require vigilant hand washing and isolation. Visitors may need to be reminded of the hospital's hand washing policies in order not to spread infection of other patients and/or visitors.

B. INFLUENZA (E.G., PANDEMIC OR EPIDEMIC)

Influenza is transmitted through large-particle respiratory droplets, such as coughing or sneezing. These droplets can travel 6 feet or less, requiring use of a mask for staff members who enter the room. Transmission may also occur through indirect contact of the hands on infected hard surfaces, so gloves must also be worn. Hand hygiene is the most important prevention intervention in transmission of influenza.

8. MULTI-ORGAN DYSFUNCTION SYNDROME (MODS)

Five stages of MODS have been identified to describe the complex process. Proinflammatory mediators that are released locally to promote wound healing at the site of injury characterize the first stage. The second stage is defined by systemic release of anti-inflammatory mediators to decrease the proinflammatory reaction. The third stage is marked by excessive systemic levels of anti-inflammatory mediators, which develop as a response to a massive proinflammatory response. The fourth stage is characterized by marked immunosuppression leaving the patient at increased risk for infection. The last stage of MODS is defined as periods of inflammation and immunosuppression.

9. MULTISYSTEM TRAUMA

Flail chest is categorized by paradoxical breathing, meaning the chest wall moves inward when the child inhales and outward when the child exhales. Extreme force, such as a blunt trauma, is the cause of flail chest. A fractured sternum (A) may lead to cardiac injury. A sucking sound when the child breathes is indicative of an open pneumothorax.

Signs and symptoms of cardiac contusion include chest pain, arrhythmias, and myocardial dysfunction. Atrial or ventricular arrhythmias are an uncommon assessment finding of cardiac contusion while S-T segment depression or elevation are more common. Management includes careful fluid administration to optimize preload, inotropic support, and manipulation of afterload with vasodilators or vasopressors.

10. PAIN

Rigid chest and abdomen are side effects of Fentanyl administration, which may require reversal with naloxone, especially if ventilation becomes difficult. Increasing vent settings may cause more damage to the child, as it does not permit more movement of the chest.

20. Which of the following patients is *most appropriate* for use of patient controlled analgesia (PCA)?
a. A 10-year-old after cardiothoracic surgery
b. A developmentally delayed 8-year-old after neurosurgery
c. A 4-year-old sickle cell patient
d. A 7-year-old with encephalopathy after a liver transplant

(See Chapter 7 for answers)

11. PALLIATIVE CARE

Palliative care is a holistic approach for patients with life-threatening or life-limiting conditions. It is not withdrawal of support, but rather total care of the patient with emphasis on management of physical and emotional pain or suffering rather than curative treatment of disease. Treatment should be managed just as aggressively as curative treatment and it requires an interdisciplinary approach as well as clear, timely communication with the family. Palliative care should be initiated as soon as a life-threatening or life-limiting illness is identified.

Palliative care seeks to improve quality of life for patients and families through prevention of physical, psychosocial, and spiritual relief and suffering. Palliative care may be implemented early in the care of patients with life-threatening illnesses. Symptom management used in palliative care improves patient outcomes and does not undermine the focus of saving the patient's life. Palliative care specialists have more time to spend with the families to identify goals and improve the patient's outcome.

12. SEPSIS CONTINUUM (SYSTEMIC INFLAMMATORY RESPONSE SYNDROME (SIRS), SEPSIS, SEVERE SEPSIS, SEPTIC SHOCK)

Sepsis/SIRS is characterized by two or more of a determined set of signs and symptoms including alteration in temperature, tachycardia/bradycardia, tachypnea, and decreased or increased leukocytes (not including neutropenia induced by chemotherapy).

13. SHOCK STATES

Shock is a complex disease process during which the tissues are not adequately perfused resulting in inadequate oxygen and nutrient supply to cells. Hypovolemic and cardiogenic shock are low-flow shock states while septic, anaphylactic, and neurogenic shock are maldistributive shock states. Complications of shock include renal failure, hepatic failure, sepsis, DIC, and death.

A. DISTRIBUTIVE (E.G., ANAPHYLACTIC, NEUROGENIC)

Anaphylactic reactions are immunoglobulin E-mediated responses resulting in rapid release of inflammatory mediators from basophils and mast cells that can lead to increased capillary permeability, vasodilatation, facial edema, bronchospasm, bronchoconstriction, and hypotension. The first-line medication used in treating anaphylaxis is subcutaneous (SQ) Epinephrine (usually dispensed in a pen). Administration of an Albuterol nebs and Benadryl are part of supportive treatment, but they are not a first-line medications.

B. HYPOVOLEMIC

Hypotensive, hypovolemic shock, requires volume replacement of 20 mL/kg of NS as the first intervention. The patient may require an epinephrine drip, administration of PRBCs, and administration of platelets, but these are not the first interventions. Two crystalloid boluses should be attempted before the patient receives any colloid replacement.

Hypovolemic shock leads to increased systemic vascular resistance as a compensatory mechanism. Early indicators of compensated hypovolemic shock include persistent tachycardia, vasoconstriction, decreased pulse pressure (the difference between systolic and diastolic blood pressure), skin mottling, prolonged capillary refill, and cool extremities.

21. A 4-year-old with hypovolemic shock and is tachycardic. The *most likely* cause is
a. Increased stroke volume caused by decreased preload and decreased cardiac output
b. Activation of peripheral and central baroreceptors causing a stream of catecholamines
c. Decreased secretion of aldosterone and antidiuretic hormone (ADH)
d. Release of microbial toxins into the bloodstream and activation of the cytokine network

(See Chapter 7 for answers)

14. SLEEP DISRUPTION (INCLUDING SENSORY OVERLOAD)

Sleep pattern disturbance and sleep apnea syndrome decreases the amount of deep sleep the patient receives and leads to changes in mood, changes in performance, fatigue, and increased irritability. During deep sleep, patients release somatostatin. Substance P is released when patients are sleep deprived, and is also noted to cause pain. When patients are chronically sleep deprived, they release less somatostatin and more substance P. Nurses should limit interruptions for care procedures and should advocate for nocturnal sleep. Nonpharmacologic and pharmacologic interventions may both be necessary.

15. SUBMERSION INJURIES

Children who have experienced drowning or submersion are at risk for hypoxic-ischemic encephalopathy, which can lead to coma, increased ICP, a vegetative state, or death. The priority immediately after drowning or submersion is aggressive resuscitation in order to prevent complications, especially prolonged hypoxia and anoxia. Hypothermic patients must be rewarmed slowly in order to prevent further cardiac compromise. Obtaining an accurate history is important to rule out abuse and/or neglect.

The most common pulmonary finding in submersion injuries is bilateral pulmonary edema. Other findings of submersion injuries include hypoxia, cerebral ischemia, atelectasis, chemical pneumonitis, pupil dilation, decerebrate posturing, decorticate posturing, seizure activity, loss of reflexes, cerebral edema, SIADH, and/or DI.

16. THERMOREGULATION

Patients at risk for thermoregulation issues include abdominal injuries, post-op cardiac surgery, post-anesthesia, burn patients, hypothyroidism, and spinal cord injury.

Patients who receive CPR immediately are typically placed on a hypothermia protocol in order to cool the patient to 32-34 degrees Celsius over 12-24 hours in order to slow down metabolism, allow the brain and heart to heal, and improve neurological outcomes. Rewarming occurs slowly at a rate of 0.3-0.5 degrees Celsius. Shivering is controlled during both cooling and rewarming phases with the use of narcotics, benzodiazepines, and neuromuscular blockers.

17. TOXIC INGESTIONS/INHALATIONS (E.G., DRUG/ ALCOHOL OVERDOSE)

Parents often feel overwhelmed with guilt, anxiety, and grief when toxic ingestion occurs at home. Family members involved in ingestion or injury are also overwhelmed with the same feelings. The whole family needs support from outside resources, such as social work. An interdisciplinary approach is vital in order to ensure that all members receive the support they need during the difficulty of an unexpected admission to the hospital.

Acetaminophen overdose causes liver toxicity and may lead to hepatic failure and death in some cases. Liver function should be monitored as frequently as every 4 hours, along with serum acetaminophen level because the liver metabolizes acetaminophen. Acetaminophen is a common poison seen because of its availability as well as its use in combination with many other medications, such as anticongestants and pain medications. It is present in over 100 household products.

Patients with acetaminophen overdose present with normal vital signs and normal mentation. Signs and symptoms include anorexia, nausea, vomiting, and right upper quadrant tenderness. Jaundice is a late finding. The antidote is N-acetylcysteine, which may be administered oral or intravenous (IV).

Clinical presentation of tricyclic antidepressant toxicity is three Cs and one A (coma, convulsions, cardiac arrhythmias, and acidosis). Early CNS symptoms include agitation, irritability, confusion, delirium, hallucinations, choreoathetosis (a combination of writhing, twisting, and contractions), seizures, and hyperpyrexia. Early cardiovascular symptoms include sinus tachycardia, hypertension, and supraventricular tachycardia (SVT).

Iron overdose causes corrosion to the GI tract. Circulating free iron injures blood vessels and hepatocytes, leading to GI bleed. Initial signs and symptoms of iron ingestion include hypotension, tachycardia, lethargy, nausea, vomiting, diarrhea, abdominal pain, and hematemesis. Symptoms of severe iron toxicity include coma, cardiovascular compromise, seizures, liver failure, and coagulopathies. When iron is metabolized, free hydrogen ions are released, producing metabolic acidosis.

Adult strength iron supplements, such as doses in prenatal vitamins, are dangerous for children under 6 years old. Iron is corrosive to the GI tract, causing absorption. Circulating free iron then injures blood vessels and damages hepatocytes. Metabolization of iron leads to release of free hydrogen and production of metabolic acidosis. The latent phase of iron intoxication occurs 2-12 hours after ingestion. Children are asymptomatic at this time, but abruptly enter the third phase, which is characterized by cardiovascular collapse.

Ingestion of the calcium channel blocker, amlodipine, leads to hypotension, reflex tachycardia, hyperglycemia, metabolic acidosis, and pulmonary edema. Conventional therapy includes calcium replacement, vasopressors, intralipids, high-dose insulin-euglycemia therapy, and plasmapheresis.

Activated charcoal absorbs many drugs and reduces the average bioavailability of drugs by 69% when given within 30 minutes of ingestion (Hazinski, 2013). However, most poison centers do not recommend its use in the prehospital setting. Administration in the emergency department may be useful if the ingestion occurred within 1 hour of presentation. Contraindications include unprotected airway, ingestion of labile substances (such as butane and other hydrocarbons), and physiological anomalies of the GI tract.

22. The nurse is caring for a toddler who has ingested an unknown number of laundry detergent packets. The nurse anticipates which of the following interventions?
a.   Placement of a nasogastric (NG) tube
b.   Administration of syrup of ipecac
c.   Initiation of a heparin drip
d.   All of the above

(See Chapter 7 for answers)

18. TOXIN/DRUG EXPOSURE (INCLUDING ALLERGIES)

Care of children with unknown drug exposure requires basic pediatric advanced life support (PALS). Subsequent care after the airway, oxygenation, ventilation, and circulation have been stabilized includes preventing further absorption of the agent. A list of drugs and chemicals in the home may be helpful in identifying the source. Physical findings that are most significant include changes in heart rate/rhythm, pupil size and reaction to light, changes in skin temperature and moisture, changes in mental status, seizures, and presence or absence of bowel sounds.

Severe symptoms of allergic reaction include dyspnea, cyanosis, difficulty speaking, tongue swelling, facial swelling, airway swelling, intense coughing, chest tightness, wheezing, stridor, laryngospasm, seizures, a sense of impending doom, hypotension, and cardiorespiratory arrest. The first intervention is to stop the causative agent, call for help, and follow PALS guidelines, which will likely include intramuscular (IM) epinephrine, diphenhydramine, albuterol nebulizer, and methylprednisolone.

Chapter 6

II. Professional Caring & Ethical Practice (20%) = 30 questions

A. ADVOCACY/MORAL AGENCY

Advocacy and moral agency are nurse characteristics in the Synergy Model in which the nurse acts on the patient's behalf to identify and help solve ethical and clinical concerns. Advocacy encompasses ethical and moral decisions based on the rights of the patient. Ensuring that informed consent is completed is part of advocacy, moral agency, and ethical nursing practice. Providing patients and families with information so they can make the best decisions about their care is the ethical duty of physicians and licensed independent providers.

B. CARING PRACTICES

Caring practices are nurse characteristics of the Synergy Model that describe activities that promote a compassionate, supportive, and therapeutic environment for patients, families, and staff members. The goal is to promote healing and comfort while reducing unnecessary suffering. Caring practices create a therapeutic environment tailored to the specific needs of the patient and family. Asking open-ended questions allows the parents to feel comfortable with the nurse and open up about their concerns and anxieties without feeling judged.

23. The nurse is caring for an infant with total anomalous pulmonary venous return (TAPVR) who remains mechanically ventilated after surgery. Which of the following is *most likely* to decrease the mother's stress level?
a.   Ensuring the child and linens are clean
b.   Asking the mother if she will be learning CPR
c.   Asking the mother if she has a support system
d.   Reviewing the child's medications

(See Chapter 7 for answers)

C. RESPONSE TO DIVERSITY

Response to diversity is a nurse characteristic in the Synergy Model defined by sensitivity to recognize, appreciate and incorporate differences into the provision of care. Differences may include, but are not limited to, individuality, cultural, spiritual, gender, race, ethnicity, lifestyle, socioeconomic, age, and values. Language barriers must be taken into account when facilitating patient and family learning.

The nurse responds to diversity by recognizing, responding to, and incorporating differences, such as language, into their practice. Differences in language can delay care, so healthcare providers must engage patients as partners in a respectful manner in order to build rapport and trust. Telephone and live medical interpreters are the only acceptable method to use when discussing updates on the patient.

D. FACILITATION OF LEARNING

Facilitation of learning by the nurse is necessary to help patients and families access health information, sort out relevant information, and adapt the information to fit their needs. Facilitation of learning is a nurse characteristic in the Synergy Model that includes both formal and informal learning. Nurses must evaluate patients who are being discharged with new equipment to ensure that the patient or the family is capable of efficiently performing tasks with the new equipment, typically with return demonstration and discussion. Nurses must also interpret informational meaning to fit the patient's and family's needs with the goal of promoting disease management at home and improving outcomes.

24. Which of the following gives the best explanation of *Clostridium difficile* to a parent?

    a. "*C. difficile* is a bacteria that may lead to malabsorption of complex carbohydrates."
    b. "*C. difficile* is a gram-positive bacteria that is acquired through contact."
    c. "*C. difficile* grows well in moist, open wounds and most frequently invades immunocompromised patients."
    d. "*C. difficile* upsets the balance of the GI tract and leads to the productions of 2 toxins that cause watery diarrhea."

E. COLLABORATION

Collaboration is a nurse characteristic that promotes patients, families, and other healthcare providers to work together to provide optimal, realistic patient/family goals. After the nursing team meets, a family meeting may be in order to identify causes of the patient's behavior as well as resolutions. Collaboration of all healthcare providers promotes each person's unique contributions to achieving optimal, realistic patient goals. Facilitation of learning by the nurse is necessary to help patients and families access health information, sort out relevant information, and adapt the information to fit their needs.

F. SYSTEMS THINKING

Systems thinking involves the nurse's knowledge and ability to navigate the healthcare environment as well as utilization of resources in the healthcare system. Systems thinking allows the nurse to review the structure, patterns, and events of a situation, rather than just the issue. The role of the nurse is to ensure that the parents feel confident and knowledgeable about emergency interventions that may be necessary after discharge in a setting outside of the hospital.

G. CLINICAL INQUIRY

Clinical inquiry is an ongoing nursing process that promotes questioning and evaluating current nursing practice in order to ensure that informed practice is being performed. The first step in clinical inquiry is collecting data in order to analyze the data, identify the problem, create an intervention, and change the current outcome. The process creates changes through evidence-based practice, research utilization, and experiential knowledge.

25. Which of the following describes the reason for enrollment gaps between eligible research participants and the number of consenting participants?
a. Lack of an available guardian
b. Disinterest of the staff
c. Lack of research staff training
d. Prolonged time collecting and analyzing data

Stephanie Doig

Chapter 7

Practice Question Answers

1. An infant exhibits bradycardia after cardiac surgery. The nurse attributes which of the following as a cause?
a. Increased systemic vascular resistance
b. Decreased pulmonary vascular resistance
c. Increased contractility
d. Decreased ventricular compliance

D. Decreased ventricular compliance
Bradycardia in an infant after cardiac surgery is often the result of decreased cardiac output. Cardiac output is a product of heart rate and stroke volume. Stroke volume is affected by preload, afterload, and contractility. Ventricular compliance is typically low immediately after cardiovascular surgery, which further affects preload and may lead to bradycardia. Increased systemic vascular resistance (A) may be a compensatory mechanism in a low cardiac state and will likely manifest as vasoconstriction and poor peripheral pulses. Decreased pulmonary vascular resistance (B) and increased contractility (C) are ideal after cardiovascular surgery in order to optimize right ventricular function and cardiac output.

2. A baby who is recovering from a patent ductus arteriosus (PDA) closure develops shortness of breath and hematuria. The nurse anticipates
a. Return to the cath lab
b. Administration of platelets
c. A portable chest x-ray

69

d. Extracorporeal membrane oxygenation (ECMO)

A. Return to the cath lab
Signs and symptoms of device migration into the aorta after PDA closure include abdominal/flank pain/distension, chest pain, shortness of breath, hematuria, decreased lower extremity pulses, or signs of decreased cardiac output and perfusion. Immediate return to the cath lab should be anticipated. Administration of platelets (B) is a temporary solution to hematuria. A portable chest x-ray (C) will show the location of the device, but is not necessary before cath lab intervention. ECMO (D) is not indicated for shortness of breath and hematuria.

3. End organ damage from dilated cardiomyopathy is caused by
a. Stiffness of the myocardium
b. Hypereosinophilic syndrome
c. Increased afterload and vasoconstriction
d. Increased release of intracellular calcium

C. Increased afterload and vasoconstriction
Dilated cardiomyopathy decreases cardiac output, decreased renal blood flow, activates the renin-angiotensin system, promotes fluid retention, causes vasoconstriction, potentiates catecholamines, stimulates the sympathetic nervous system, increases heart rate, and increases contractility. Vasoconstriction to the vital organs occurs at the sacrifice of increased afterload (C). Stiffness of the myocardium (A) and hypereosinophilic syndrome (B) are the results of restrictive cardiomyopathy. Increased release of intracellular calcium (D) is a function of hypertrophic cardiomyopathy.

4. Assessment findings of a patient's electrocardiogram (ECG) reveal a heart rate of 124 bpm with an inverted P-wave immediately following each R-wave. The nurse anticipates which of the following?
a. Initiation of overdrive pacing
b. Synchronized cardioversion
c. Administration of potassium chloride
d. Administration of packed red blood cells

A.   Initiation of overdrive pacing
Accelerated junctional rhythm is an arrhythmia associated with postop cardiac surgery. It is characterized by a regular, fast heart rate (120-200 bpm) with P-waves that are often hidden in the QRS, but may also come immediately after the R-wave and will be inverted in leads II, III, and AVF. The beat coming from the AV node (instead of from the sinus node) results in loss of atrial kick. Loss of atrial kick is especially detrimental after cardiac surgery. Inverted P-waves are the result of retrograde electrical activity from the AV node up to the atria. Treatment includes pacing, antiarrhythmics, and treatment of underlying conditions. The metabolic rate can be decreased through cooling measures, paralyzation, and sedation.

5. A child is noted to have a prolonged PR interval. The nurse suspects which of the following as the cause?
a. Systemic lupus erythmatosus
b. ASD closure
c. Hypermagnesemia
d. Hypoglycemia

D. Hypoglycemia

Causes of first-degree heart block include hypoglycemia, digoxin, calcium channel blockers, beta-blockers, sotalol, rheumatic heart disease, Lyme disease, myocarditis, muscular dystrophy, hypokalemia, hyperkalemia, hypocalcemia, hypercalcemia, and hypomagnesemia (C). Systemic lupus erythmatosus (A) and ASD closure (B) may lead to third-degree heart block.

6. The knee-to-chest position is appropriate treatment of cyanosis in which of the following patients?
a. Unrepaired congenital mitral stenosis
b. Unrepaired tetralogy of Fallot
c. Unrepaired AV canal
d. Unrepaired hypoplastic left heart syndrome

B. Unrepaired tetralogy of Fallot
Tetralogy of Fallot is a cyanotic heart defect with four anomalies including a ventricular septal defect (VSD), right ventricular outflow obstruction, an overriding aorta arising from the VSD, and right ventricular hypertrophy. Hypoxemic "tet" spells are thought to be caused by transient increase in right ventricular outflow obstruction, decreased systemic vascular resistance, decreased pulmonary blood flow, and increased right to left shunting. Mitral valve stenosis (A) is an obstructive defect presenting with congenital heart failure symptoms. AV canal (C) is an acyanotic defect. Hypoplastic left heart syndrome (D) is an obstructive defect treated with staged palliative surgeries.

7. The function of surfactant is to
a. Vasodilate the pulmonary vasculature
b. Decrease pulmonary shunting

c. Decrease viscosity of pulmonary secretions
d. Prevent alveolar collapse at end expiration

D. Prevent alveolar collapse at end expiration

Surfactant is a slick, soapy substance secreted by type II pneumatocytes in the alveoli that prevents alveolar collapse at end expiration. Surfactant is decreased in premature infants leading to respiratory distress syndrome. Surfactant administration in premature infants leads to increased lung compliance by decreasing the surface tension at the air-liquid interface of the alveoli. It is not a vasodilator (A), nor does it affect pulmonary shunting (B). Viscosity of pulmonary secretions are not affected by surfactant (D).

8. Interpret the following blood gas
    pH 7.50
    CO2 32 mmHg
    HCO3 31 mmol/L
    pO2 87
   a. Respiratory acidosis
   b. Respiratory alkalosis
   c. Metabolic acidosis
   d. Metabolic alkalosis

D. Metabolic alkalosis

The pH is high (normal is 7.35-7.45), the pCO2 is low (normal is 35-45 mmHg), the bicarbonate is high (normal is 24-28 mmol/L), and pO2 is low (which does not affect acid/base balance). Metabolic alkalosis is the result of a loss of acid or a gain of bicarbonate. Bicarbonate can be gained in the presence of hypochloremia, hypokalemia, of after diuretic therapy with inadequate electrolyte replacement. Metabolic alkalosis may also result from excessive administration of sodium bicarbonate.

9. The nurse expects which of the following blood gas results in a child with a central nervous system disorder?
   a. Respiratory acidosis
   b. Respiratory alkalosis
   c. Metabolic acidosis
   d. Metabolic alkalosis

B. Respiratory alkalosis

Primary respiratory alkalosis is rare in children. Respiratory alkalosis is the result of central nervous system disorders, drug toxicity, salicylate poisoning, advanced liver failure, or emotional hyperventilation. Respiratory acidosis (A) results from inadequate respiratory drive, such as intrinsic airway disease, chest all instability, a compromised diaphragm, compromised upper airway muscle function, or alveolar disease. Metabolic acidosis (C) results from oxidation of fatty acids (such as in DKA or salicylate poisoning), lactic acid production, or accumulation of inorganic acids. Metabolic alkalosis (D) may result from hypochloremia, hypokalemia, diuretic therapy, or excessive administration of sodium bicarbonate.

10. A patient with diabetes insipidus exhibits polyuria. The *most likely* reason is
a. High serum blood glucose levels

b. Low antidiuretic hormone levels
c. High urine osmolality
d. Low serum sodium levels

B. Low antidiuretic hormone levels
Diabetes insipidus (DI) is classified by a lack of antidiuretic hormone (ADH) and is treated with ADH replacement with Desmopressin (also called DDAVP). DI affects blood glucose levels (A). Urine osmolality is low (C) (< 200 mOsm/kg) and serum sodium (> 145 mEq/L) is high (D) in DI due to a decrease in both urine concentrating ability and water conservation resulting in excessive diuresis.

11. A patient with acute lymphoblastic leukemia (ALL) is on a norepinephrine drip for septic shock after induction chemotherapy 2 days prior. The last set of laboratory findings are as follows:

Potassium	5.9 mEq/L
Phosphorus	4.9 mg/dL
Calcium	7.8 mg/dL
BUN	7.5 mmol/L

The nurse anticipates which of the following interventions?
a. Vigorous IV hydration
b. Increasing the norepinephrine drip
c. Administration of Kayexalate
d. Administration of IV calcium chloride

A.   Vigorous IV hydration
Tumor lysis syndrome (TLS) is a potentially life-threatening oncologic complication that can lead to acute renal failure (ARF). It usually occurs after effective chemotherapy or radiation therapy, but it can also occur after treatment with glucocorticoids, antiestrogen

tamoxifen, and interferon. TLS leads to rapid release of intracellular metabolites that exceeds the capability of the kidneys to excrete. Potential effects include hyperuricemia, hypocalcemia, hyperphosphatemia, and hyperkalemia. Treatment of TLS is prevention with vigorous hydration and allopurinol before cancer treatment.

12. Sickle cell disease is suspected in an 8-year-old. Diagnostic findings consistent with this diagnosis include
a. Abnormal peripheral blood smear and anemia
b. Positive blood cultures and hyperglycemia
c. Elevated aspartate aminotransferase (AST) and alanine aminotransferase (ALT)
d. Leukocytosis and bandemia

A. Abnormal peripheral blood smear and anemia
Diagnostic findings for a sickle cell patient include a peripheral blood smear with sickled cells. A complete blood count (CBC) shows anemia because the spleen has destroyed the sickled cells. Bilirubin may be elevated due to hemolysis of the sickled cells. A chest x-ray may show cardiomegaly and pulmonary infiltrate with acute chest syndrome. A computed tomography (CT) scan and/or magnetic resonance imaging (MRI) are indicated if cerebrovascular accident (CVA) is suspected.

13. Octreotide may be used in the treatment of which patient?
a. Rotavirus infection
b. Hyperbilirubinemia
c. Hemorrhagic pancreatitis
d. Ascites

C. Hemorrhagic pancreatitis

Causes of hemorrhagic pancreatitis may be obstructive, nonobstructive, or inflammatory. Signs and symptoms include Cullen's sign (a bluish discoloration around the umbilicus) and Turner's sign (bluish discoloration in the flanks. Rotavirus infection is treated with IV fluids (A). Phototherapy is typically used to treat hyperbilirubinemia (B). Treatment of ascites (D) includes identifying and correcting the cause of ascites to prevent respiratory compromise.

14. A child develops tachycardia on postop day 5 after abdominal surgery. The nurse's next action is to

a. Perform pulmonary hygiene
b. Administer rectal acetaminophen
c. Inspect the abdominal incision
d. Assess bilateral lung sounds

C. Inspect the abdominal incision

Tachycardia and fever on postoperative day 5 is likely infectious, such as from a wound (C). A fever on postoperative days 1-3 is most likely noninfectious, such as atelectasis, which would validate suctioning, oral care, incentive spirometry, or other pulmonary hygiene (A). Evaluation of the wound must occur before administration of antipyretics (B). A wound infection is more likely to be the cause of than atelectasis making assessment of the wound a priority over assessing lung sounds (D).

15. The nurse is admitting a child with chronic kidney disease (CKD). The nurse should assess which of the following *first*?

a. Sodium level
b. Blood glucose level
c. Blood urea nitrogen (BUN)
d. Hemoglobin level

A. Sodium level
Initial assessment of a child with CKD includes evaluation of serum electrolytes. Renal damage decreases the ability of the kidneys to concentrate urine. Sodium and water restrictions may result in hyponatremia while children with end-stage renal disease are unable to excrete sufficient amounts of sodium resulting in hypernatremia. Hypervolemia may be an indication for dialysis or continuous renal replacement therapy (CRRT).

16. The nurse is caring for a child with acute renal failure. The nurse expects which of the following assessment findings?
a. Hypernatremia
b. Hypercalcemia
c. Hyperkalemia
d. Hypophosphatemia

C. Hyperkalemia
Injury to the distal tubules impairs the ability of the kidneys to excrete potassium-causing hyperkalemia. Acute renal injury may be caused by hypovolemia, hypotension, shock, renal artery thrombosis, or aortic thrombosis. Laboratory findings include metabolic acidosis, hyperkalemia, hyponatremia (A), hypocalcemia (B), hyperphosphatemia (D), hyperuricemia, and hypermagnesemia.

17. A child receiving negative pressure wound therapy (NPWT) to a deep sternal wound infection after cardiac surgery has saturated the foam dressing and filled the drainage container 3 hours after the dressing was changed. The *first* intervention by the nurse is to
a. Notify the licensed independent practitioner (LIP)
b. Replace it with a wet to dry sterile dressing
c. Contact the wound ostomy continence nurse (WOCN)
d. Quantify and document the amount of blood loss

A. Notify the licensed independent practitioner (LIP)
Complications of NPWT include bleeding, infection, and retained dressing material. Children receiving NPWT for deep sternal wounds are at risk for bleeding from the capillaries, native arteries, native veins, vascular grafts, and the right ventricle. Bleeding is most often the result of mechanical injury. The dressing should be replaced with a wet to dry sterile dressing (B) temporarily if the device is malfunctioning. The WOCN will likely be contacted (C) and the amount of blood loss will need to be quantified and documented (D), but the source of excessive bleeding must be identified and controlled first.

18. A 3-week-old is awaiting brain death testing. The mother tells the nurse she is sure the baby cannot be brain dead because she sees the baby's feet move when she touches the leg. The nurse's best response is

a. "These movements are likely spinal cord reflexes, which are reflexes of the spinal cord that run from the feet to the spinal cord and back."

b. "Your baby still has spinal cord reflexes, which may continue despite cerebral cortex injury and brain death."

c. "We will have to wait to see the results of the brain death testing to determine from where the movement is being generated."

d. "The movement that you're seeing is not considered purposeful movement, such as tracking with the eyes, sucking, or grasping an object."

A. "These movements are likely spinal cord reflexes, which are reflexes of the spinal cord that run from the feet to the spinal cord and back."

Spinal cord reflexes do not require involvement of the higher levels of the central nervous system (CNS), therefore spinal cord reflexes may be present even in a child who is clinically brain dead. Discussing the cerebral cortex injury (B) and explaining purposeful movement (D) are likely too technical for parents, especially for parents in distress. Telling the parents they will have to wait for the brain death testing results (C) increases the mother's anxiety.

19. A school-aged child recovering from arteriovenous (AV) malformation repair begins to experience emesis, headache, and altered mental status. The *most likely* cause is
a. Brainstem herniation
b. Encephalopathy
c. Cerebrovascular accident
d. Diabetes insipidus

C. Cerebrovascular accident
AVM is an abnormal communication between arteries and veins without an interposed capillary bed. Cerebrovascular accident (CVA) may be ischemic or hemorrhagic in nature. Hemorrhagic CVA may result from small arteries damaged by hypertension,

rupture of aneurysms, rupture of arteriovenous malformation, bleeding disorders, or cocaine abuse. Desired outcomes in treatment of AVM include no hemorrhage, no rebleeding, and no vasospasm.

20. Which of the following patients is *most appropriate* for use of patient controlled analgesia (PCA)?
a. A 10-year-old after cardiothoracic surgery
b. A developmentally delayed 8-year-old after neurosurgery
c. A 4-year-old sickle cell patient
d. A 7-year-old with encephalopathy after a liver transplant

A. A 10-year-old after cardiothoracic surgery
PCAs are used in alert, oriented (D), developmentally appropriate (B) school-aged children (C) or older. Cardiothoracic postoperative pain may be more efficiently managed with use of a PCA than traditional pain control with as-needed analgesics if the patient and family are properly educated on use. Inadequate treatment of postop pain may lead to the child forming a "pain memory", as well as risk of experiencing chronic pain which can result in long-term physical, psychological, social, and developmental effects (Epstein, 2017).

21. A 4-year-old is in the PICU with hypovolemic shock and is tachycardic. The *most likely* cause is
a. Increased stroke volume caused by decreased preload and decreased cardiac output
b. Activation of peripheral and central baroreceptors causing a stream of catecholamines
c. Decreased secretion of aldosterone and antidiuretic hormone (ADH)
d. Release of microbial toxins into the bloodstream and activation of the cytokine network

B. Activation of peripheral and central baroreceptors causing a stream of catecholamines

Hypovolemia is the most common cause of shock in infants and children. It causes a decrease in preload that reduces stroke volume and cardiac output (A). Activation of the renin-angiotensin-aldosterone system promotes the release of aldosterone increasing the kidney's reabsorption of sodium (C). ADH is released as an additional compensatory mechanism to promote reabsorption of sodium. Release of microbial toxins into the bloodstream and activation of the cytokine network (D) is consistent with septic shock.

22. The nurse is caring for a toddler who has ingested an unknown number of laundry detergent packets. The nurse anticipates which of the following interventions?
a. Placement of a nasogastric (NG) tube
b. Administration of syrup of ipecac
c. Initiation of a heparin drip
d. All of the above

A. Placement of a nasogastric (NG) tube
Toddlers are at risk of ingesting detergent packets due to their draw to small, colorful objects. Treatment is supportive and includes gastric decompression with an NG tube. Clinical effects include respiratory compromise, lethargy, nausea, vomiting, diarrhea, mucosal damage, and metabolic acidosis. Administration of syrup of ipecac (B) and initiation of a heparin drip (C) are not indicated.

23. The nurse is caring for an infant with total anomalous pulmonary venous return (TAPVR) who remains mechanically ventilated after

surgery. Which of the following is *most likely* to decrease the mother's stress level?
a. Ensuring the child and linens are clean
b. Asking the mother if she will be learning CPR
c. Asking the mother if she has a support system
d. Reviewing the child's medications

A. Ensuring the child and linens are clean
Mothers of children with congenital heart defects are at increased risk for stress after cardiac surgery. Infant appearance and behavior was identified as the biggest stressor, followed by sights and sounds (Lisanti, Ryan Allen, Kelly, & Medoff-Cooper, 2017). CPR can be discussed when the child is preparing for discharge (B). Asking about the mother's support system (C) and reviewing the child's medications do not address the immediate concerns she may have regarding the way the infant appears and whether or not the child appears to be in pain.

24. Which of the following gives the best explanation of *Clostridium difficile* to a parent?

a. "*C. difficile* is a bacteria that may lead to malabsorption of complex carbohydrates."

b. "*C. difficile* is a gram-positive bacteria that is acquired through contact."

c. "*C. difficile* grows well in moist, open wounds and most frequently invades immunocompromised patients."

d. "*C. difficile* upsets the balance of the GI tract and leads to the productions of 2 toxins that cause watery diarrhea."

D. "*C. difficile* upsets the balance of the GI tract and leads to the productions of 2 toxins that cause watery diarrhea."

Antibiotic therapy can change the microbial ecology of the GI tract, leading to a decrease in normal intestinal flora, proliferation of toxins A and B, amplification of toxins A and B, and secretory diarrhea. It is a gram-negative, spore-producing bacteria. Rotavirus may lead to malabsorption of complex carbohydrates (A). *Staphylococcus aureus* and *staphylococcus epidermidis* are gram-positive bacteria that are acquired through contact (B). *Pseudomonas aeruginosa* is an opportunistic organism that grows well in moist, open wounds (C).

25. Which of the following describes the reason for enrollment gaps between eligible research participants and the number of consenting participants?
    a. Lack of an available guardian
    b. Disinterest of the staff
    c. Lack of research staff training
    d. Prolonged time collecting and analyzing data

A. Lack of an available guardian
Nurses should be engaged in clinical inquiry development to improve patient outcomes. Gaps in research enrollment have been attributed to lack of an available legal guardian (A), limited enrollment time, limited availability of research staff, family dynamics, and language barriers. Research participants must meet the inclusion criteria and have an available guardian to sign consent (if the patient is a minor) during the enrollment period in order to participate. Families may feel too overwhelmed with the patient's illness to agree to participate.

References

Adler, J. (2014). Therapeutic Hypothermia. Available at: http://emedicine.medscape.com/article/812407-overview

Andersson Mattox, E. (2017). Reducing Risks Associated with Negative-Pressure Wound Therapy: Strategies for Clinical Practice. *Critical Care Nurse, 37*(5). 66-67. doi: https://doi.org/10.4037/ccn2017308

American Heart Association. (2010). *Guidelines for Cardiopulmonary Resuscitation and Emergency Cardiovascular Care Science.* Available at: http://circ.ahajournals.org/content/122/18_suppl_3.toc.

Bettencourt, A. & Mullen, J. E. (2017). Delirium in Children: Identification, Prevention, and Management. *Critical Care Nurse, 37*(3). E9-e18. doi:https://doi.org/10.4037/ccn2017692

Centers for Disease Control and Prevention, Division of Birth Defects, National Center on Birth Defects and Developmental Disabilities. (2016). Autism Spectrum Disorder (ASD): Facts About ASD [Data file]. Retrieved from http://www.cdc.gov/ncbddd/autism/facts.html

Centers for Disease Control and Prevention, National Center for Emerging and Zoonotic Infectious Diseases (NCEZID), Division of Healthcare Quality Promotion (DHQP). (2016). *Healthcare-Associated Infections: Carbapenem-resistant Enterobacteriaceae in Healthcare Settings.* Retrieved from http://www.cdc.gov/HAI/organisms/cre/

Centers for Disease Control and Prevention, National Center for Immunization and Respiratory Diseases (NCIRD). (2016). *Influenza: Prevention Strategies for Seasonal Influenza in Healthcare Settings.* Retrieved from http://www.cdc.gov/flu/professionals/infectioncontrol/healthcaresettings.htm

Centers for Disease Control and Prevention, National Center for Injury Prevention and Control, Division of Violence Prevention. (2016). *Child Abuse and Neglect: Prevention Strategies* [Data file]. Retrieved from http://www.cdc.gov/violenceprevention/childmaltreatment/prevention.html

Curley, M. A. (2007). Synergy: *The Unique Relationship Between Nurses and Patients.* Indianapolis, IN: Sigma Theta Tau.

Epstein, H.M. (2017). Postoperative Patient-Controlled Analgesia in the Pediatric Cardiac Intensive Care Unit. *Critical Care Nurse, 37*(1). 55-61. doi: https://doi.org/10.4037/ccn2017724

Hardin, S. R. & Kaplow, R. (eds.). (2005). *Synergy for Clinical Excellence: The AACN Synergy Model for Patient Care.* Sudbury, MA: Jones & Bartlett.

Hazinski, M. F. (2013). *Nursing Care of the Critically Ill Child.* 3rd ed. St. Louis, MO: Mosby/Elsevier.

Lisanti, A.J., Ryan Allen, L., Kelly, L., & Medoff-Cooper, B. (2017). Maternal Stress and Anxiety in the Pediatric Cardiac Intensive Care Unit. *American Journal of Critical Care, 26*(2). doi:https://doi.org10.4037.ajcc2017266

Kerfoot, K.M., Lavandero, R., Cox, M., Triola, N., Pacini, C., & Hanson, M.D. (2006). Conceptual models and the nursing organization. *Nurse Leader, 4*(4), 20-26.

Mathiesen, C., McPherson, D., Ordway, C., & Smith, M. (2015). Caring for Patients Treated with Hypothermia. *Critical Care Nurse, 35*(5), e1-e12. Doi 10.4037/ccn2015168

Mayo Clinic. (2017). Osteomyelitis. Retrieved from https://www.mayoclinic.org/diseases-conditions/osteomyelitis/basics/definition/con-20025518

Meningitis Now. (n.d.). Types and Causes [Data file]. Retrieved from https://www.meningitisnow.org/meningitis-explained/what-meningitis/types-and-causes/

National Library of Medicine. (2015). *Inborn errors of metabolism*. Retrieved from https://medlineplus.gov/ency/article/002438.htm

Pasek, T. A., Geyser, A., Sidoni, M., Harris, P., Warner, J. A., Spence, A., . . . Weicheck, S. (2008). Skin Care Team in the Pediatric Intensive Care Unit: A Model for Excellence. *Critical Care Nurse, 28*(2). 125-135. http://ccn.aacnjournals.org/content/28/2/125.full.pdf

Perrin, K.O. & Kazanowski, M. (2015). Overcoming Barriers to Palliative Care Consultation. *Critical Care Nurse, 35*(5). 44-52.

Rauen, C. (2016). Certification Test Prep: Life Can Get in the Way Sometimes. *Critical Care Nurse, 36*(4). 76-79. doi: http://dx.doi.org/10.4037/ccn2016235

Rauen, C., Jeffries, K., Flynn Makic, M. B. (2016). Certification Test Prep: We Do It for Our Patients. *Critical Care Nurse, 36*(2). 74-77. doi: http://dx.doi.org/10.4037/ccn2016791

Rauen, C., Gendron-Trainer, N., & Muller, M. L. (2015). Certification Test Prep: The Devil Is in the Details. *Critical Care Nurse, 35*(5). 68-72.

Rauen, C., Knippa, S., & Clark, C. (2017). Certification Test Prep: This Is the Year to Listen to Yourself. *Critical Care Nurse, 37*(1). 70-74.

Rauen, C., Tollefson, T., & Dietzler, H. (2016). Certification Test Prep: Certification: A Credential of Competence. *Critical Care Nurse, 36*(1). 80-83.

Reuter-Rice, K. E. & Peterson, B. M. (2016). Conventional and Unconventional Lifesaving Therapies in an Adolescent With Amlodipine Ingestion. *Critical Care Nurse, 36*(4). 64-49. doi: http://dx.doi.org/10.4037/ccn2016524

Saleem, A. F., Ariff, S., Aslam, N., & Ikram, M. (2010). Congenital Bilateral Choanal Atresia. Journal of the Pakistan Medical Association, 60(10). 869-872.

http://www.academia.edu/535221/Case_Report_Congenital_Bilateral_Choanal_Atresia

Selekman, J. & Jakubik, L. D. (2014). *Pediatric Nursing Certification Review* (3rd edition). Chicago, IL: Society of Pediatric Nurses. https://www.practicequiz.com/question/15215/D?sub_token=6425e8207ee29278bcd9b8260900959b43b38094

Siegrist Thomas, J. (2016). Certification Test Prep. *Critical Care Nurse, 36*(3). 66-70. Professional Caring and Ethical Practice

Slota, M.C. (2006). Core Curriculum for Pediatric *Critical Care Nursing* (2nd ed.). St Louis, MO: Saunders Elsevier.

Soeholm H., Kirkegaard H. (2014). Serum Potassium Changes During Therapeutic Hypothermia After Out-of-Hospital Cardiac Arrest-Should It Be Treated? *Therapeutic Hypothermia Temperature Management*, 2(1). 30-6. doi: 10.1089/ther.2012.0004.

Sole, M.L., Middleton, A., Deaton, L., Bennett, M., Talbert, S., & Penoyer, D. (2017). Enrollment Challenges in Critical Care Nursing Research. *American Journal of Critical Care, 26*(5). doi:https://doi.org10.4037.ajcc2017511

Stanford Children's Health. (2017). *Failure to Thrive*. Retrieved from http://www.stanfordchildrens.org/en/topic/default?id=failure-to-thrive-90-P02297

Urden, L., Stacy, K., & Lough, M. (2014). *Critical Care Nursing: Diagnosis and Management* (7th ed.). St Louis, MO: Elsevier Mosby.

Wilson Shah, L. (2016). Ingestion of Laundry Detergent Packets in Children. *Critical Care Nurse, 36*(4). 70-75. doi: http://dx.doi.org/10.4037/ccn2016233